THE CARE AND FEEDING
OF AN ——
IACUC

The Organization and Management
of an Institutional Animal Care
and Use Committee

Edited by

M. Lawrence Podolsky, M.D.
Victor S. Lukas, D.V.M.

CRC Press

Boca Raton London New York Washington, D.C.

St. Petersburg
Junior College

Library of Congress Cataloging-in-Publication Data

The care and feeding of an institutional animal care and use committee
/ edited by M. Lawrence Podolsky, Victor S. Lukas.
      p.   cm.
    Includes bibliographical references (p.   ) and index.
    ISBN 0-8493-2580-3 (alk. paper)
    1. Animal welfare. 2. Animal rights. 3. Animals--Treatment.
4. Laboratory animals--Moral and ethical aspects. I. Podolsky, M.
Lawrence. II. Lukas, Victor S.
HV4708.C35 1999
179′.4—dc21
                                        98-51623
                                          CIP

© 1999 by CRC Press LLC

No claim to original U.S. Government works
International Standard Book Number 0-8493-2580-3
Library of Congress Card Number 98-51623
Printed in the United States of America 1 2 3 4 5 6 7 8 9 0
Printed on acid-free paper

Foreword

The framers of the 1985 amendments to the Federal Animal Welfare Act (AWA) envisioned the Institutional Animal Care and Use Committee (IACUC) as the linchpin—the central and cohesive element—of the laboratory animal care and use program at research, education, and testing organizations. Effective operation of this committee is essential if these organizations are to achieve full regulatory compliance, and, more importantly, retain the public's support for activities involving the use of animal subjects.

In 1987, the Scientists Center for Animal Welfare, in cooperation with the American Association for Laboratory Animal Science, published a compilation of presentations made at five regional workshops on effective operation of IACUCs (Orlans, F. B., Simmonds, R. C., and Dodds, W. J., Effective Animal Care and Use Committees, *Lab. Anim. Sci.*, Special Issue, 1987). In the decade since this compilation was published, nearly all of the 18 consensus recommendations developed by the workshop participants and the Center's Board of Trustees have either been incorporated into the AWA regulations (e.g., committee members should be appointed by the highest institutional official) or have been voluntarily adopted by institutions using animal subjects (e.g., use of a system to categorize experiments based on their level of ethical concern). *The Care and Feeding of an IACUC* superbly illustrates the progress and advances the animal-using communities have made in implementing these and other improvements in their animal care and use programs.

The highly qualified contributors provide 12 information-packed chapters and 10 exceptionally helpful appendixes that should provide researchers, administrators, and IACUC chairs and members with an indispensable reference volume. This book summarizes information critically necessary for the effective and efficient management and operation of an IACUC, and as such should be made available to IACUC members and administrative officials in every institution using laboratory animals.

Richard C. Simmonds, D.V.M., M.S., ACLAM
Diplomate Director, Laboratory Animal Medicine
University and Community College System of Nevada

Reno, Nevada

The Editors

M. Lawrence Podolsky, B.A., M.D., F.A.A.P received his medical degree from The University of Health Sciences/Chicago Medical School in 1945. Following his internship and postgraduate training at Baylor Medical School, Houston, TX, Sea View Hospital, Staten Island, NY, and at La Rabida Sanitorium, Chicago, IL, he was certified by the American Board of Pediatrics in 1955 and became a Fellow of the American Academy of Pediatrics in 1960. For many years, as a member of the Pediatric Academy's Indian Health Committee, he was an activist for better health care for Alaskan and American Indians. He has held academic research and teaching appointments at the University of Chicago, Stanford University, and the Children's Hospital of Baylor Medical College. His past and present memberships include the American Medical Association, California Medical Association, San Mateo County Medical Society, the American College of Chest Physicians, and the American Association for the History of Medicine.

He was a captain in the U.S. Army and attended the Medical Field Service School at Fort Sam Houston, TX. Most of his military life was spent as Chief of Medicine and Pediatrics at the U.S. Army Hospital in Baumholder, Germany.

In addition to extensive medical, pedagogic, and writing activities, he has held numerous civic and political offices. He served as mayor, councilman, planning commissioner, environmental officer, and chairman of the Noise Abatement Committee in the city of Belmont. From 1967 to 1972 he served on the San Francisco Bay Area Air Pollution Control District both as a member of the board of directors and as a member of its Science Advisory Council. He also was a member of the San Mateo County Environmental Quality Control Commission. He engaged in civic improvement work as a member of the Lions Club and flew with Flying Samaritans to bring medical help to Indians in remote parts of the United States and Mexico.

He currently serves on a committee that regulates and monitors experimentation on humans in Veterans Administration hospitals and acts as a consultant to the pharmaceutical industry on the organization and operation of institutional animal care and use committees.

During his transition from medical practice to popular writing in the early 1970s, he took creative and technical writing courses at the College of San Mateo and the University of California at Berkeley. In 1977 he was elected to membership in the American Society of Journalists and Authors and has served as one of its directors. In August 1989, he received an Award of Excellence in Journalism from the American College of Emergency Physicians. He authored the book *Cures Out of Chaos,* which was published in 1998, and has had over 200 articles published in professional journals and popular magazines.

For relaxation he fly fishes, sails, and raises bonsai trees.

Victor S. Lukas, D.V.M., is a Department Head of Veterinary Services and the Cell Culture Core Facility at Roche Bioscience in Palo Alto, CA. He has been a member of the Roche Bioscience Institutional Animal Care and Use Committee for 12 years and currently serves as chair from 1995 to 1998.

Dr. Lukas received his B.S. in 1975 and his Doctor of Veterinary Medicine degree in 1977 from Michigan State University in East Lansing, MI. Upon graduation, he served as a veterinarian in the Peace Corps for two years on the island of Grenada, West Indies. When he returned to the United States, he was employed for two years as a large animal veterinarian in private practice in Michigan. In 1981, he began his career in research while employed at Laboratory Animal Research Enterprises in Kalamazoo, MI. In 1983, Dr. Lukas entered the NIH Postdoctoral Fellowship Program in Laboratory Animal Medicine at The University of Michigan Medical School in Ann Arbor, MI. Upon completion, he was employed as a Veterinary Medical Officer at the Palo Alto Veterans Administration Medical Center. He was board certified in 1987 by the American College of Laboratory Animal Medicine and also began employment at Syntex Research, Palo Alto, CA which later became Roche Bioscience. He has served on the Board of Directors for the Santa Clara Valley Science and Engineering Fair and the Children's Preschool Center in Palo Alto, CA.

Contributors

Paula Belloni, Ph.D.
Principal Scientist
Roche Bioscience
Palo Alto, CA

Joanne R. Blum, D.V.M.
Diplomate, American College
  of Laboratory Animal Medicine
Principal
Advanced Bioresources Inc.
San Jose, CA

Michael D. Kreger, M.S.
Technical Information Specialist
Animal Welfare Information Center
National Agricultural Library
Beltsville, MD

Victor S. Lukas, D.V.M.
Diplomate, American College
  of Laboratory Animal Medicine
Department Head, Veterinary Services
Roche Bioscience
Palo Alto, CA

M. Lawrence Podolsky, M.D.
IACUC member
Roche Bioscience
Palo Alto, CA
Protein Design Labs, Inc.
Mt. View, CA
California Pacific Medical Center
  Research Institute
San Francisco, CA

Stephen P. Schiffer, D.V.M., M.S.
Diplomate American College of
  Veterinary Internal Medicine and
  American College of Laboratory
  Animal Medicine
Director
Division of Comparative Medicine
Associate Professor of Cell Biology,
Georgetown University
  Medical Center
Washington, D.C.

Richard C. Simmonds, D.V.M., M.S.
Diplomate, American College of
  Laboratory Animal
  Medicine
Director, Laboratory Animal
  Medicine
University and Community
  College System of Nevada
Reno, NV

Philip C. Tillman, D.V.M.
Diplomate, American College
  of Laboratory Animal Medicine
Campus Veterinarian
University of California
Davis, CA

Robert J. Tressler, Ph.D.
Associate Director of Pharmacology
CHIRON Corporation
Emeryville, CA

Sonja L. Wallace, A.A.S., R.V.T.
Research Supervisor
Veterinary Services
Chair of IACUC Training Subcommittee
Roche Bioscience
Palo Alto, CA

Sally K. Wixson, V.M.D. M.S.
Diplomate, American College
  of Laboratory Animal
  Medicine
Director, Animal Resources
BASF Bioresearch Corporation
Worcester, MA

Introduction

The federal government's concern about the welfare of animals began in 1873, when Congress passed the Twenty-Eight-Hour Law stipulating that animals en route to markets had to be rested and watered at least every 28 hours. But thereafter, for almost an entire century, animals were generally ignored.

In July 1965, a Dalmatian named Pepper disappeared from her backyard. She was traced to an animal dealer and then to a research laboratory, where she had been euthanized. Pet owners demanded reprisals. Because there were no laws in effect at that time to curb such practices, no crime had been committed and nothing could be done. A storm of protests flooded the media. Animal owners, Washington's Animal Welfare Institute (AWI), New York and Pennsylvania state police, and local officials were galvanized into a force that demanded legislative action. In response, New York Congressman Resnick introduced a bill that required dog and cat dealers, and laboratories that purchased them, to be licensed and inspected by the U.S. Department of Agriculture. The bill also mandated that animals were to be handled in accordance with humane standards established by the Secretary of Agriculture. Similar legislation was introduced into the Senate by Warren Magnusen and Joseph Clark. Research laboratories and laboratory animals were initially exempted—in response to heated opposition to the bills—but they were restored again under an amendment sponsored by Senator Mike Monroney. Finally, the bills were passed by the House and Senate and signed into law by President Johnson on August 24, 1966. This became known as the 1966 Laboratory Animal Welfare Act. It vested regulatory authority in the Secretary of the U.S. Department of Agriculture (USDA), who was to implement it through the USDA's Animal and Plant Health Inspection Service (APHIS), Veterinary Services (later named Regulatory Enforcement and Animal Care (REAC), which was shortened to Animal Care). In 1970, the act was renamed the Animal Welfare Act, or AWA.

The 1966 Act applied to only six species of animals. Their coverage ceased once they were assigned to a research protocol. In 1970, all warm-blooded vertebrates (with some exclusions) were covered during their entire stay at an institution. Dealers were required to become licensed and registered, transport standards were introduced, and exhibitors were brought under regulation. An amendment in 1976 brought carriers under regulation.

The next major event occurred in December 1985, when Congress added the Dole-Brown amendments to the omnibus Farm Bill—called the Improved Standards for Laboratory Animals—which, as stated by Senator Dole, were designed to minimize pain and distress to laboratory animals. In effect, however, the amendments, plus the bill as a whole, made the federal government directly responsible for the supervision and regulation of the use of animals in all educational and research institutions as well as by breeders, transporters, and exhibitors of animals.

On March 15, 1989, the U.S. Department of Agriculture published in the *Federal Register* 132 triple-columned pages of text that spelled out the conditions that would go into effect with the new law. Prior to that, from 1985 until the publication of the final regulations in 1989, the USDA asked for and received almost 36,000 comments on the proposed regulations. These ranged from demands for far more stringent regulations to requests for no new regulations at all. The nation as a whole, however, favored improved standards in the laboratory.

The new legislation mandated the establishment of IACUCs, or Institutional Animal Care and Use Committees. Earlier, however, both The Health Research Extension Act of 1985 (PL99-158) and the 1986 Public Health Service (PHS) Policy on Humane Care and Use of Laboratory Animals had also established Institutional Animal Care and Use Committees. More than a thousand IACUCs were already functioning in 1989, the time when the regulations of the Animal Welfare Act were adopted. Whereas the former legislation spelled out IACUC responsibilities in institutions where PHS projects were funded, the Animal Welfare Act empowered IACUCs to approve or disapprove the use of animals for all experimental and teaching purposes. IACUCs were also charged with overseeing the training of personnel in research facilities, inspecting animal housing to enforce approved standards of hygiene and comfort of animals, and making sure that animals were treated humanely and received pain-relieving drugs whenever necessary.

The voluminous directives in the *Federal Register* initially incited widespread fear and confusion among those who depended upon animals for their livelihood, education, or research. The latter were particularly dismayed when it became apparent that all funding for research conducted or supported by any component of the Public Health Service depended upon complying with these directives.* The financial impact was also intimidating. To set up the program, universities, corporations, and research facilities faced one-time capital costs of $876 million and another $207 million in annual operating expenses (see Horton). Early on, some research was contracted out to facilities in Europe and Russia, but it returned to the United States when other countries subsequently adopted regulations patterned on American standards.

The Animal Welfare Act did not, perhaps could not, spell out exactly how IACUCs were to carry out their duties and responsibilities. Back then, no one could envision the extended use of animals in outer space or the impacts of cloning, transgenic animals, the proliferation of mono- and polyclonal antibody production, microsurgeries, transplants, xenotransplants/xenografts, embryonic manipulations, and other emerging technologies. Hence, no guidelines could be formulated in PHS policy or in USDA regulations. Additionally, situations encountered by universities differed from those in the pharmaceutical industry, and these in turn differed from facilities where teaching or cosmetic testing was the primary pursuit. To their credit, IACUCs all over the nation faced these new, unexpected challenges as they arose, and developed the consensus of attitudes and practices that provide today's guiding

---

* Toward the end of 1995 USDA-APHIS, FDA, and NIH renewed their memorandum of understanding whereby each agency, under its own authority, assumed responsibilities for assuring proper animal care and welfare.

principles—which, incidentally, have been incorporated into periodic USDA updates and adopted by other nations.

Now, with more than a decade of experience behind them, educators and researchers have, more or less, come to terms with IACUCs and the new regulations. Moreover, they have established operating procedures that assure compliance with the law without otherwise constraining initiatives and progress. It is the intent of this book to succinctly present that hard-earned wisdom, and in so doing, pave the way for cordial relationships between animal users, accrediting agencies, the government, and society.

The title of this book, *The Care and Feeding of an IACUC,* may seem whimsical; nevertheless, it points to important factors that contribute to the efficiency and effectiveness of IACUCs. They must have *Care* in order to maintain critical evaluations of their practices, for without care they could easily drown in lethargy. As for *Feeding,* they must constantly forage through the fonts of knowledge and imbibe new developments and advanced information if they are to act as the intermediary between science, the regulators, and the voiceless animal.

Inasmuch as many members of IACUCs may be students or other people with little or no scientific or technical knowledge, the authors, wherever possible, have reduced technical terms to a minimum and presented thoughts and data in the simplest language. Our ultimate goals are, first, to provide useful, practical information, or references to such material, that IACUC members at all levels of scientific comprehension can put to use; and second, to find ways to say *Yes!*—to show how IACUCs can carry out their responsibilities without unduly interrupting research.

Some topics have been repeated or restated in several chapters—record keeping, inspections, assessing pain in animals, roles of the veterinarian, and guides formulated by other organizations or agencies such as AAALAC (Association for Assessment and Accreditation of Laboratory Animal Care, International) and the NIH (National Institutes of Health). This was necessary to allow for the presentation of different viewpoints on the same subject; it also made the chapters more comprehensive.

This book augments many of the discretionary elements of the Animal Welfare Act. It neither replaces the Animal Welfare Act nor serves as a substitute for the rules, regulations, and policies of the U.S. Department of Agriculture. It is incumbent upon all institutional officials and investigators to keep abreast of modifications and revisions of the law, and policies of enforcement agencies, as they change to accommodate new concepts and advanced technologies.

V. S. L.

M. L. P.

REFERENCE

Horton, L., Commentary: the enduring animal issue, *J. Nat. Cancer Inst.,* 81(10), 736, 1989.

Acknowledgments

We thank James Woody, M.D., Ph.D., President, Roche Bioscience, Palo Alto, CA, for making corporate resources available to the authors. Martin Sidor, D.V.M., M.S., Director, Bioservices, Roche Bioscience, and Daniel Ringler, D.V.M., Professor and Director of the Department of Laboratory Animal Medicine, University of Michigan Medical School, suggested topics for coverage, read the manuscript, and made significant editorial improvements. Chuck Bullock and Sigmund T. Rich, D.V.M. of Protein Design Laboratories and Greg Stickrod of California Pacific Medical Center Research Institute, proffered much practical information and valuable advice, predicated on their many years of experience as directors and coordinators of IACUC activities. Jean A. Larson, M.A., Coordinator, Cynthia Smith, M.S., Tim Allen, and Richard Crawford, D.V.M., Technical Information Specialists, all with the Animal Welfare Information Center, contributed substantive material and constructive ideas for Chapter 11, The Literature Search for Alternatives. Lilla Nickerson, BASF Bioresearch, provided invaluable administrative and editorial assistance to Chapter 9. Deborah L. Jacobstein, Information Scientist, Library and Information Center, Roche Bioscience, reviewed all sources for literature searches and provided valuable corrections and augmentations. Nancy Mize and Debra Benkelman, Roche Bioscience, provided much needed computer and administrative assistance.

Contents

Chapter 1

M. Lawrence Podolsky, M.D.

Chapter 2

M. Lawrence Podolsky, M.D.

Chapter 3

Philip C. Tillman, D.V.M.

Chapter 4

Stephen P. Schiffer, D.V.M., M.S.

Chapter 5

M. Lawrence Podolsky, M.D.

Chapter 6

Victor S. Lukas, D.V.M.

Chapter 7

Sonja L. Wallace, A.A.S., R.V.T.

1 IACUC: The Hub of Communication

M. Lawrence Podolsky, M.D.

CONTENTS

IACUCs may vary in their individual operations, but they all direct their efforts toward a common purpose: to make sure that the animals under their purview are used and cared for in a humane manner. Essentially, they serve as animal research ethics boards committed to the welfare of animals.

As intermediaries between science and the public, IACUCs must judge the merits of the research carried out at their facility. As intermediaries between science and the law, they must enforce the policies and regulations of the Animal Welfare Act.* To carry out this mission:

- IACUCs are responsible for reviewing, at least every six months, their institution's program for the humane care and use of animals. Their evaluations, reports, and recommendations regarding the research facilities, animal use, and personnel training programs are sent to the chief executive officer, dean, or similar institutional official.
- At least once every six months, IACUCs inspect all animal facilities, including those off-site, for compliance with approved standards for hygiene and comfort of animals, and report findings to the institutional official. These reports identify departures from regulations or standards and state reasons, if any; they distinguish significant from minor deficiencies; and they provide for a plan and schedule for corrections. Inasmuch as everyone might not agree on the criteria for acceptance or disapproval, both majority and minority opinions may become part of such reports.

---

* Many IACUCs take into account the Public Health Service Policy on Humane Care and Use of Laboratory Animals, the National Institutes of Health (NIH) Guide for the Care and Use of Laboratory Animals, and the recommendations of the Association for Assessment and Accreditation of Laboratory Animal Care. They also develop their own additional policies and guidelines for institutional laboratory animal resources.

TABLE 1.1
Federally Mandated IACUC Functions

1. Review, at least once every six months, the research facility's program using the USDA Regulations/ *Guide* as basis.
2. Inspect, at least once every six months, all of the animal facilities including animal study areas/satellite facilities, using the USDA Regulations/*Guide* as basis.
3. Prepare reports of IACUC evaluations and submit the reports to the Institutional Official.
4. Review and investigate legitimate concerns involving the care and use of animals at the research facility resulting from public complaints and from reports of noncompliance received from facility personnel or employees.
5. Make recommendations to the Institutional Official regarding any aspect of the research facility's animal program, facilities, or personnel training.
6. Review and approve, require modifications in (to secure approval), or withhold approval of those components of proposed activities related to the care and use of animals.
7. Review and approve, require modifications in (to secure approval), or withhold approval of proposed significant changes regarding the care and use of animals in ongoing activities.
8. Suspend an activity involving animals when necessary, take corrective action, and report to the funding agency and the USDA.

- IACUCs review and approve, require modifications, or withhold approval of all protocols for the use of animals in teaching and research.
- IACUCs review and approve, require modifications, or withhold approval of changes and amendments to protocols.
- IACUCs oversee the training of personnel involved in the care or use of animals.
- IACUCs make sure that animals are provided with proper husbandry and veterinary care, receive pain relieving drugs, and require justification for using death as an endpoint.
- IACUCs suspend an activity involving animals whenever necessary. They take corrective action and report findings and actions to all appropriate funding agencies and the U.S. Department of Agriculture (USDA).
- IACUCs review and investigate reports of noncompliance with the law or questionable practices or procedures. Complaints may come from a facility, personnel, employees, or the public.*

See Table 1.1.

1.1   CONTINUING REVIEW

Public Health Service policy, as well as the animal welfare regulations of the USDA, requires IACUCs to review all ongoing research, testing, teaching, training, and

---

*Complaints are made on an Animal Incident form that assures anonymity. IACUCs may investigate directly or ask a subcommittee to verify the allegation before the matter is presented to the full IACUC. Complainants may make inquiries about findings, actions, and dispositions. See Chapter 4 for more on this.

related activities not less than once every three years. Most IACUCs adhere to the admittedly more stringent Animal Welfare Act regulations and conduct reviews on an annual basis rather than triennially. This can be done either as a committee of the whole or by using a designated reviewer process.

These reviews are designed to:

1. Inform the IACUC of the current status of projects.
2. Ensure continued compliance with the Public Health Service (PHS), the USDA, and institutional requirements.
3. Provide for reevaluation of all animal activities at appropriate intervals.

They must address pain and distress, pain relief, animal husbandry, veterinary care, personnel qualification, and methods of euthanasia.

Factors to be considered at every review include:

- Current status of the project—investigators should supply information on the funding status, number of animals used, and proposed amendments. Some IACUCs insist on a statement about the progress being made in achieving the specific aims of the protocol.
- Compliance with PHS, USDA, and institutional requirements—investigators should provide assurances that the animal activity has not deviated (or provide an explanation if it has changed) from the approved protocol and that protocols comply with changing standards. Protocols, even after approval by the IACUC, may have to be revised by the principal investigator to clarify certain sections, for example, animal numbers in the design may add up to less than the number requested, or methods of anesthesia and euthanasia seem questionable. Perhaps the foremost reason behind a request for revision is to take into account new advanced technologies or new *in vitro* techniques, which, if implemented, would lead to reductions in the number of animals used, refinements in procedures that assure less pain and suffering, and perhaps, the replacement of mammals by invertebrates or nonanimal insentient modalities.
- Ethical cost–benefit analysis—IACUCs must evaluate animal pain, morbidity, and mortality against the potential benefits of the project in terms of its relevance to human or animal health, advancement of knowledge, or the good of society. IACUCs should take this opportunity to reevaluate their approval criteria and/or to modify their rules and standards. Note, however, that "merit" review is not required by USDA or PHS, although it could be required by institutional policy.

The entire IACUC membership should receive a copy of completed continuing review forms. These forms are described in the next chapter.

1.2 HUB OF COMMUNICATION

Perhaps the most understated yet most important function of an IACUC is to serve as the hub of communication (Figure 1.1). This communication may be direct, but more

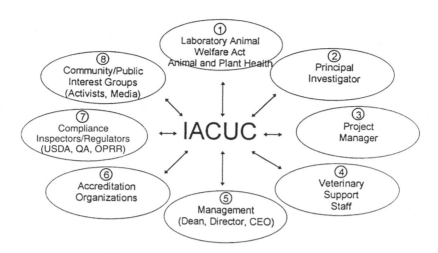

FIGURE 1.1   The IACUC is the hub of communications.

often, it is voiced by the attending veterinarian (AV), the IACUC chair and staff, and the institutional official.

1.   *The Law*—IACUCs try to carry out both the letter and spirit of the law as stated in the Animal Welfare Act and in PHS Policy. Avenues of communication exist in both directions to accommodate ever-changing circumstances, the emergence of new technologies, and to iron out controversies and differences in interpretations of specific directives.

IACUCs keep abreast of the changes and modifications of the law. The Act, since 1966, focused on improving animal care and use in research, teaching, and testing. When amended in 1985, it included psychological well-being for nonhuman primates and exercise in dogs. It is now incumbent for IACUCs to make such enrichments part of their considerations.

When U.S.D.A. Policy 12 was implemented and full text was sent to everyone covered by AWA, W. Ron DeHaven, Acting Deputy Administrator, Animal Care, USDA, made it patently clear in his September 1997 health report that IACUCs could no longer assume that researchers had carried out good-faith searches for alternatives. "Our policy," he stated, "is based on a federal mandate to avoid or minimize discomfort, distress, and pain. It includes the expectation that principal investigators will not simply stop searching if they do not find a nonanimal model. Instead, we would expect the concepts of refinement and reduction to be applied wherever possible in order to minimize animal pain/distress when it cannot be eliminated. While Congress did not intend to eliminate animals in research, they clearly did intend to minimize pain and distress, a fact that is especially evident in the 1985 amendment to the Act." It is now incumbent upon IACUCs to scrutinize all protocols for adequate narrative by principal investigators that documents the literature search for alternatives and to vote for approval only when satisfied that the search was comprehensive and carried out "in good faith." See Chapter 11.

The most recent change in thinking to affect IACUCs appeared in November 1997, when the National Institutes of Health, Office for Protection from Research Risks (OPRR), stated that "there is evidence that the mouse ascites method of monoclonal antibody production causes discomfort, distress, or pain. Practical *in vitro* methods exist which can replace the ascites method in many experimental applications without compromising the aims of the study.

Accordingly, IACUCs are expected to critically evaluate the proposed use of the mouse ascites method. Prior to approval of proposals that include the mouse ascites method, IACUCs must determine that:

1. The proposed use is scientifically justified.
2. Methods that avoid or minimize discomfort, distress, and pain (including *in vitro* methods) have been considered.
3. The latter have been found unsuitable.

Fulfillment of this three-part IACUC responsibility, with appropriate documentation, is considered central to an institution's compliance with its Animal Welfare Assurance and the PHS Policy." (See Reference 2.)

The standards adopted by the signers of the European Convention for the Protection of Vertebrate Animals Used for Experimental and other Scientific Purposes to some extent are more stringent than those in the United States. These standards are gradually being adopted by some American IACUCs. The European Convention, for example, considers monoclonal antibody production (MAb) *in vitro* as the norm, while the mouse ascites method may be used only when it has been proven that it is the only way to attain specific diagnostic or therapeutic products. This concept is not yet entrenched in the United States but may be an indicator of where we are headed.

2. *Principal investigator*—IACUCs are the main link to the principal investigator (see Chapters 6 and 11 on protocols and rapport with researchers), and assist in devising experiments that reduce pain and suffering of animals while reducing the number of animals used. Indeed, IACUCs are the best advocates for the three R's: replace existing animal methods with nonanimal methods whenever possible, reduce the number of animals needed, and refine research procedures to minimize pain and discomfort. (See Sources at the end of this chapter and in Appendices for detailed information on testing alternatives.)

3. *Project managers*—IACUCs consult with project managers so that all plans for research or development of animal models comply with USDA regulations before they go into effect. It is not uncommon for the IACUC, Radiation Safety Committee, and the Biosafety Committee to be involved in a single project. Rapid and concise communications between these bodies is essential for the reduction and elimination of corporate or bureaucratic drag.

4. *Veterinary support*—IACUCs lean heavily on veterinarians and staff for advice about animals and for training purposes. Veterinarians, on the other hand, need input from IACUCs, especially from public and outside members, to properly assess complaints and criticisms about animal handling, ethics, and the relevancy of proposed research.

5. *Management*—Deans, CEOs, and corporate and institutional officials are directly responsible for all research and the proper use of animals within their organizations. They must, of necessity, rely upon the IACUC's semiannual reviews of ongoing research, inspections of animal facilities, and self-evaluations in order to find out where deficiencies exist and then eliminate or correct them. Strong upper-level support of IACUCs is essential.

6. *Accreditation organizations*—IACUCs may need to cooperate with AAALAC and all other accrediting organizations. Accreditation depends upon proper IACUC organization and function. (A review of AAALAC's *Description of the Animal Care and Use Program,* plus updates and revisions, could be included in IACUC's semiannual program reviews.)

7. *Inspections/compliance*—Inspections by federal agencies focus primarily on the physical plant that houses animals, IACUC meeting minutes, and content of protocols and their methods of execution. When the IACUC performs well, inspectors seldom find a fault.

8. *Community and the public interest*—IACUCs are essentially windows to the world. In addition to placing outside, nonaffiliated members on IACUCs, IACUC meetings at nonprivate institutions may be open to the public and the media. Wherever this was challenged, court orders usually granted public access to IACUC meetings. Indeed, in Washington state, where Sunshine Laws are in effect, IACUC meetings may be held amidst cameras and a gallery of spectators. In government funded universities it is not unusual for students to attend IACUC meetings. In any event, IACUCs must be prepared to defend their reasoning and actions at any meeting, public or private. All committee members must ask themselves, "If the experiment I am about to approve makes headlines on the front pages of tomorrow's newspapers, could I justify my action?" (See Tillman, Chapter 3, and Schiffer, Chapter 4 for other perspectives on this subject.)

SOURCES AND SUGGESTED READING

1. Russell, W. M. S. and Burch, R. L., *The Principles of Humane Experimental Techniques,* Metheun & Co., London, 1959. (Reprinted as a special edition in 1992 by the Universities Federation for Animal Welfare.)
2. Gary, B., Ellis, G. B., and Garnet, N. L. P., *AWIC Newsletter,* Winter 1997/1998, Vol. 8, No. 3-4.
3. Public Health Service (IV.C.1.a), Public Health Service Policy on Humane Care and Use of Laboratory Animals, U.S. Department of Health and Human Services, Washington, D.C. 1986.
4. U.S. Government, Principles for the Utilization and Care of Vertebrate Animals Used in Testing, Research, and Training, Development by IRAC and endorsed by the Public Health Service Policy on Humane Care and Use of Laboratory Animals, 1985.
5. U. S. Government Principles for the Utilization and Care of Vertebrate Animals Used in Testing, Research, and Training, Principle II, OPRR, Bethesda, MD, 1986.
6. Animal Welfare Regulations, Code of Federal Regulations, Title 9 (Animals and Animal Subprojects), Subchapter A (Animal Welfare), Section 2.31(e)(4).
6a. International Guiding Principles, Biomedical Research Involving Animals, developed by the Council for International Organizations of Medical Sciences, Switzerland, 1985.

7. Animal Testing Alternatives (Partial list; see Chapter 11 for comprehensive guides.), The Humane Society of the United States (HSUS), the Center for Alternatives to Animal Testing (CAAT) at the Johns Hopkins University School of Public Health, The Procter & Gamble Company, the National Institutes of Health Office for Protection from Research Risks (OPRR), the U.S. Department of Agriculture Animal Welfare Information Center (AWIC) and Animal and Plant Health Inspection Service (APHIS), the Food and Drug Administration Office of Science, and Utrecht University, The Netherlands, have formed a coalition to promote a website designed to increase access to information on ways to implement the three R's. It can be accessed on the Internet at http://infonet.welch.jhu.edu/~caat. For more information contact The Procter & Gamble Company, (513) 945-8039, or Johns Hopkins Center for Alternatives to Animal Testing, (410) 995-3343.

A full bibliography with abstracts on *Alternatives to the Use of Live Vertebrates in Biomedical Research and Testing* is available from the Toxicology and Environmental Health Information Program, Specialized Information Services, National Library of Medicine, National Institutes of Health, Bethesda, MD.

8. Boschert, K., IACUCs and the World Wide Web, *Lab Animal,* 26(5), 38, 1997.

2 Formation and Composition of an IACUC

M. Lawrence Podolsky, M.D.

CONTENTS

An IACUC, as defined in the Animal Welfare Act, must have at least a chairperson and two other members—a veterinarian and an outside, nonaffiliated public member. The Public Health Service (PHS) Policy on Humane Care and Use of Laboratory Animals, 1986, specifies that an IACUC shall consist of not less than five members: one doctor of veterinary medicine, one scientist, one nonscientist, and at least one outside member who is not a user of animals and is not affiliated with the institution. The validity of IACUC actions is always based on a properly constituted IACUC.

A recent survey* revealed that IACUCs ranged from 3 to 50 members, with the median being 7 voting members. Of those IACUCs that responded to the survey, 90 percent had fewer than 14 members. Appointments were made by the dean, CEO, or other official of the institution directly responsible for the program.

Commonly, more than the minimum number of members are appointed. By so doing, such problems as absenteeism and lack of a quorum are reduced or eliminated. Some institutions have made it a policy to rotate their members on a regular basis, such as every two to three years. While this has the advantage of infusing the committee with new blood and new thinking, it also results in the loss of much valuable knowledge and experience acquired by long-standing memberships. Also, time is wasted introducing novices to the basics of IACUC operations.

---

* Scientists Center for Animal Welfare (SCAW) engaged Cygnus Corporation, a survey company, to carry out a national IACUC survey to provide information and data on how IACUCs carry out their responsibilities. Survey packets were mailed to 1200 institutions on January 31, 1996.

0-8493-2580-3/99/$0.00+$.50
© 1999 by CRC Press LLC

Another option is to appoint nonvoting members. These are individuals with expertise in various fields who can explain highly technical matters to the committee and suggest appropriate courses of action. In IACUCs on which I have served, I was especially appreciative of having engineers, architects, hazardous waste material handlers, building maintenance people, heat and light technicians, and similar experts on hand to explain, even simplify, situations not completely understood by the IACUC as a whole.

Veterinarians are the linchpins of the IACUC. By virtue of education and experience, they can tell whether the animal listed in the protocol is best suited for the designated usage, whether it is experiencing pain and distress, and when euthanasia is indicated.

Scientists may be principal investigators, biologists, physicists, chemists, division heads, or other science faculty. These members can understand some of the more esoteric complexities involved in a protocol and explain them to other members of the IACUC.

Nonscientists often include members of the legal, business, and administrative staffs who can make judgments on the legal and financial ramifications of a protocol. Other disciplines include librarians, animal care specialists, members of the clergy, and the liberal arts faculty.

Outside members may include clergy, students, lay people, teachers, physicians, skilled and nonskilled workers, elected officials, and attorneys (unaffiliated with the school or company)—for that matter, any responsible person in the community.

2.1 SPECIAL CONSIDERATIONS

While the addition of active or retired clergy, lawyers, and judges may add prestige to an IACUC, this advantage is often offset by the need to educate and train people unfamiliar with the language and nature of science. Long debates, with votes based on built-in biases rather than on fact, may waste inordinate amounts of time at IACUC meetings.

In academic settings, students, either individually or through student government, and faculty regard appointments to IACUCs as a way to participate in the affairs of the institution. The advantage of including students is that they are young and are in a position to inspire new ideas. The disadvantage may lie in their insistence upon the ideal rather than on the feasible.

In the nonscientist category, it is advisable to enroll architects, engineers, health and safety officers, building maintenance personnel, quality assurance people, supervisors and managers of animal facilities, and other specialists familiar with the design, construction, operations, and maintenance of animal facilities.

The outside member category may include anyone listed in the nonscientist category or anyone in the community. Often, the best compromise, in my opinion, is found in retired science teachers and retired physicians, because they already have a basic understanding of science and a maturity that enables them to weigh ethical issues against the potential value of research.

2.2   COMPENSATION

As a rule, employees of a university, pharmaceutical company, or governmental institution receive no additional compensation for serving on IACUCs. Such service is considered a normal extension of their employment. Outside members, on the other hand, are generally compensated for their time and travel expenses. The amount they receive varies widely. Some are paid per meeting, others receive an annual retainer. Reimbursement rates are also affected by the frequency of meetings, the number of protocols reviewed, and the budgets of individual organizations. In any case, reimbursements should not be overly generous in order to avoid the perception that such compensation influences opinions and decisions. Additional perks include snacks, drinks, free lunch, preferential parking, and, of course, expanded knowledge. No federal funds are available for compensating IACUC members.

2.3   NONVOTING MEMBERS

The size of IACUCs generally ranges from 7 to 14 members. A small size offers the advantages of quick decisions and little expense. However, this reduces the amount of expertise available to the committee and thereby limits input and debate. A very large IACUC can be unwieldy, hard to assemble a quorum, and may be costly. One way to get around this problem is to appoint nonvoting members to the IACUC. Experts in law, engineering, architecture, transportation, health and safety, and other disciplines that touch upon the work of IACUCs can find a useful niche for their talents without encumbering the IACUC with added size and additional expense.

In-house statisticians and information specialists, who assist investigators in developing study protocols and literature searches, may also serve as ex officio members of an IACUC. There is no limit to the number of nonvoting members that may be affiliated with an IACUC.

2.4   IACUC GUIDE

Although there is no legal requirement to do so, it is a good idea for every IACUC to prepare a notebook or similar reference source that documents its authority, defines its purpose, establishes its position within the corporation or academic institution, and compiles, in one place, all of the rules, policies, and guidelines that have been adopted from time to time. (See Chapter 7, The IACUC's Role in Education and Training, for detailed coverage of this subject.)

Ideally, the IACUC should make rules and policies that serve as guides for investigators and administrators. These rules and policies should implement the law faithfully, address identifiable problems, act in the public interest, be consistent with other rules and policies (federal, state, and international), and should be based on adequate information and be rationally justified. Additionally, they should accomplish goals cost-effectively and should be easily understood. In essence, they should be acceptable and enforceable and stay in effect only as long as necessary.

SOURCES AND SUGGESTED READING

Animal Welfare Information Center (AWIC), *Animal Welfare Information Center Newsletter,* National Agricultural Library, AWIC, 10301 Baltimore Avenue, Beltsville, MD 20705, NAL call number AHV4701.A952. This newsletter covers a wide range of topics relevant to the scientific community and the IACUC. Topics include animal welfare regulations, Animal Care and Use Committees, agricultural animal care, alternatives, legislation updates, upcoming meeting, funding sources, new AWIC products and services, and scientific and general articles on animal care and use issues and methods. Subscriptions are free. Back issues are available on the AWIC website: http://www.nal.usda.gov/awic.

Berry, D., Reference materials for members of animal care and use committees, National Agricultural Library, Animal Welfare Information Center, Beltsville, MD, NAL call number aHv4701.A95 no. 10, 1991. Annotated bibliography of books and proceedings about animal care and use committees covering 1977 to 1991.

Canadian Council on Animal Care, Animal care committees: role and responsibilities, Canadian Council on Animal Care, Ottawa, ON, Canada, NAL call number HV4708 A55, 1992. Proceedings from a workshop sponsored by the Canadian Council on Animal Care (CCAC) in February 1992. Topics include researcher responsibilities, ethical concerns, psychology protocol reviews, media concerns, CCAC Alternatives Committee, peer review, occupational health and safety, training personnel, monitoring field studies, invertebrates, and workshop reports.

Canadian Federation of Humane Societies, *Guidelines for Lay Members of Animal Care Committees,* Canadian Federation of Humane Societies, Nepean, ON, NAL call number HV4735.G8, 1986. Describes the functions and activities of animal care committees; includes sections entitled "Lay committee members: special people with special problems," "How to review protocols," and "Pain."

Council of the Applied Research Ethics National Association (ARENA), *Institutional Animal Care and Use Committee Guidebook,* National Institutes of Health Publication No. 92-3415, National Institutes of Health, Bethesda, MD, NAL call number HV4764.158, 1992. Excellent overview of Institutional Animal Care and Use Committee composition, function, proposal review, oversight of the animal care and use program, record keeping, sample forms, and special considerations; useful review of NIH policies and the Animal Welfare Act as they pertain to the committee.

Code of Federal Regulations (CFR), Title 9 (Animals and Animal Products), Subchapter A (Animal Welfare), Office of the Federal Register, Washington, D.C., 1985.

Editorial Committee of Institutional Administrators and Laboratory Animal Specialists for the Henry M. Jackson Foundation for Advancement of Military Medicine, Uniformed Services University of Health Sciences, *Institutional Administrator's Manual for Laboratory Animal Care and Use,* U.S. Department of Health and Human Services, Public Health Service, National Institutes of Health, Bethesda, MD, NAL call number SF406 154, 1988. Available from the Office for Protection from Research Risks, National Institutes of Health, 6100 Executive Boulevard, Suite B01, Rockville, MD 20892-7507. A guide for institutional administrators who supervise laboratory animal care and use programs. The manual addresses questions involving quality care, ethics, and legal requirements for animal care and use programs.

Guttman, H. N., Mench, J. A., and Simmonds, R. C., Eds. *Science and Animals: Addressing Contemporary Issues,* Scientists Center for Animal Welfare, Greenbelt, MD, NAL call number HV4704.S33, 1989. Proceedings from a conference held by the Scientists Center for Animal Welfare in 1988. "Community and lay members of animal care and use committees," "Animal care and use committee issues," and "Well-being and ethics" are three of the six sections contained in this volume. The community and lay member session was developed and presented entirely by active community and lay members of Animal Care and Use Committees.

Johns Hopkins University, School of Hygiene and Public Health, Animal care and use committees and alternatives, symposium sponsored by the Johns Hopkins School of Hygiene and Public Health, Office for Research Subjects, Johns Hopkins Center for alternatives to animal testing, Baltimore, MD, NAL call number HV4704.A53, June 18, 1992. Transcript of lectures about the concept of alternatives, their use in science, information resources, regulatory requirements, and IACUC involvement in precollege education.

Krulisch, L. The SCAW IACUC survey: preliminary results, *Lab. Animal,* 26(5), 28, 1997.

Laboratory Animal Science Association and Universities Federation for Animal Welfare, *Guidelines on the Care of Laboratory Animals and Their Use for Scientific Purposes.* IV—*Planning and Design of Experiments,* Ennisfield, London, England, NAL call number SF406.G8 v.4, 1990. Basic recommendations as to the planning and design of experiments using animals, and how this can affect the outcome of the experiment.

National Institutes of Health, Office of Protection from Research Risks, NIH Office of Animal Care and Use, *Animal Care and Use: Policy Issues in the 1990s,* Office of Animal Care and Use, National Institutes of Health, Bethesda, MD, NAL call number HV4704.A46, 1989. Proceedings from the NIH OPRR/OACU conference, November 16–17, 1989, Bethesda, MD.

National Institutes of Health Animal Research Committee, *Using Animals in Intramural Research: Guidelines for Investigators and Guidelines for Animal Users,* NIH Office of Animal Care and Use, Bethesda, MD, NAL call number HV4928.U85, 1994. NIH Research Advisory Committee notebook outlining the NIH IACUC program, occupational safety, laws and regulations, ethical and scientific issues, alternatives, pain and distress.

National Research Council (NRC), *Guide for the Care and Use of Laboratory Animals,* National Academy Press, Washington, D.C., 1996.

Orlans, F. B., Research Protocol review for animal welfare, *Invest. Radiol.,* 22, 253, 1987. An overview of protocol review, investigators' concerns about IACUCs, and assessing and minimizing animal pain and distress.

Orlans, F. B., *Field Research Guidelines: Impact on Animal Care and Use Committees,* Scientists Center for Animal Welfare; Greenbelt, MD, NAL call number HV4704.F5, 1988. The proceedings of a workshop entitled "Field Research Standards" held on October 8, 1987.

Orlans, F. B., Simmonds, R. C., and Dodds, W. J., Eds. *Effective Animal Care and Use Committees, Laboratory Animal Science, Special Issue,* Scientists Center for Animal Welfare, Golden Triangle Building One, 7833 Walker Drive, Suite 340, Greenbelt, MD 20770, email: scaw@erols.com. NAL call number 410.9P94, 1987. Papers from workshops sponsored by the Scientists Center for Animal Welfare focusing on effective review of biomedical experiments to ensure humane and appropriate use of animals. Includes chapters concerning the objectives and activities of animal care and use committees, protocol review and animal pain, and roles of committee members, including lay members.

Public Health Service (PHS), Public Health Service Policy on Humane Care and Use of Laboratory Animals, U.S. Department of Health and Human Services, (PL 99-158, Health Research Extension Act, 1985), Washington, D.C., 1996.

Public Responsibility in Medicine and Research (PRIM&R) and Tufts University School of Medicine, *Animal Care and Use Programs: Regulatory Compliance and Education in an*

Age of Fiscal Constraint, PRIM&R, Boston, MA, NAL call number HV4913.A54, 1991. Educational material for animal care and use programs.

Scientists Center for Animal Welfare (SCAW), *SCAW Newsletter,* Golden Triangle Building One, 7833 Walker Drive, Suite 340, Greenbelt, MD 20770, tel: (301) 345-3500, fax: (301) 345-3503, number QL55.N48. Quarterly newsletter that promotes the humane treatment of animals used in research. Articles frequently focus on animal care and use committees.

Theran, P. The SCAW IACUC survey: the unaffiliated member, *Lab. Animal,* 26(5), 31, 1997.

U.S. Department of Agriculture, Directive 635.1, Humane Care and Use, Agricultural Research Service, Washington, D.C., NAL call number aKF3841.D57, 1990. Description of requirements for animal care and animal care and use protocols for use by the USDA, Agricultural Research Service researchers and veterinary staff.

U.S. Department of Defense, Report to the Senate Armed Services Committee and the House of Representatives National Security Committee on Department of Defense Animal Care and Use Programs, Department of Defense, Washington, D.C., NAL call number HV4928.U56, 1995. The fiscal year 1995 report to Congress on the Department of Defense animal care and use programs in research, education, and training for defense and extramural projects.

University of Texas Health Science Center at San Antonio, *Responsible Care and Use of Animals in Research and Training,* Institutional Animal Care Training Program, San Antonio, TX, NAL call number HV4933.T4U5, 1990. Description of the university's program, relevant legislation, alternatives, organization resources, zoonoses, facilities, and animal health management.

3 IACUC Records and Their Management

Philip C. Tillman, D.V.M.

CONTENTS

0-8493-2580-3/99/$0.00+$.50
© 1999 by CRC Press LLC

3.1   FUNDAMENTALS VS. OVERHEAD

Research institutions acquire new knowledge and disseminate that knowledge. When a research facility gains new scientific knowledge, develops a new drug, publishes an article in a scientific journal, or trains a new physician, it acts in accord with its primary mission. When a research facility performs a maintenance activity, satisfies a regulatory requirement, or pursues any activity other than research and teaching, it engages in an overhead activity.

Some Facilities and Administration (F&A) activities, also called overhead activities, are necessary. Institutions must keep the offices warm and safe, pave their parking lots, and keep the toilets in their bathrooms functioning; but such F&A/overhead activities are not the fundamental purpose of a university. We perform a good service for our institutions and society when we minimize the amount of time and money spent on overhead activities.

Record keeping is an F&A/overhead activity. Writing records, filing them, retrieving them, refiling them, and disposing of them is a constant and usually a nonproductive chore. Although records are necessary, we should strive to reduce the amount of time and resources devoted to them. Our greatest efforts, as IACUC members, should be devoted to direct animal care and to assisting scientists with the conduct of their research and teaching.

3.2   WHO NEEDS THIS RECORD?

I cannot imagine a year passing without someone, either within or outside the institution, suggesting that some additional form or revised record should be generated and stored. Such requests should be viewed with skepticism and resisted where possible. Ask yourself, "Who will use this record?" The answer will place the record in one of two categories, which I call internal records and mandated records.

3.2.1   INTERNAL RECORDS

If it is not an outside body, but an employee who requests the record, then it is an internal record. If an employee steps forward and declares that he or she wants and needs the information, will cherish the record, care for it, and use it regularly, then by all means generate the record. The employee or unit that needs and uses the record should be the one who maintains it. If the record is not externally mandated, and exists entirely for internal purposes, it may take any form we choose. We can keep it as long as we need it and then discard it when we are done with it.

3.2.2   MANDATED RECORDS

If the record is mandated by an external body, many aspects of our record keeping will be dictated by the agency requiring the record. Examples of mandated records

TABLE 3.1
IACUC Records Mandated by PHS Policy as Described in PHS Animal Welfare Policy Sections IV.E. and IV.F.

Record	Recipient	Frequency	Retention	Comment
Animal Welfare Assurance	A mutually acceptable document must be negotiated between the institution and OPRR	A new Animal Welfare Assurance must be filed every five years	Keep the currently approved version of the document at all times. Older versions may be discarded	OPRR requires that this document be made available to all investigators
Annual report to OPRR	OPRR	Once yearly	Three years	Must include any minority views
Reports of semiannual evaluation of programs and facilities	Institutional official	Twice yearly	Three years	Must include minority views
Protocols and amendments of protocols	The IACUC itself	Whenever such documents are submitted or acted upon	Three years after cessation of the activity	The IACUC must also issue "Letters of Verification" for proposals as evidence of IACUC approval
Accrediting Body Determinations (such as of AAALAC site visits)	From AAALAC to the institutional official	Whenever such correspondence is received (at least every three years)	Three years	AAALAC will not make their documents public, but if the accredited institution is a public entity, then it will be required to make its AAALAC correspondence public
Prompt reporting documents— reports of serious or continuing deficiencies, deviations from the guide, or suspensions of activities by the IACUC	OPRR	Promptly, whenever such incidents occur	Three years	Must include any minority views

Note: Tables 3.1 and 3.2 are not intended to be complete listings of all the records a facility might want to keep (or be required to keep). Research institutions are obliged to keep large numbers of records dealing with diverse matters such as Occupational Health and Safety, controlled substances, exotic species, training, accreditation, driver safety, good laboratory practices, and so forth. These tables are limited to records needed to prove compliance with the USDA regulations or PHS Animal Welfare Policy.

TABLE 3.2
IACUC Records Mandated by USDA Regulations as Described in
9 CFR Subpart A, Sections 2.35 and 2.31

Record	Recipient	Frequency	Retention	Comment
Minutes of IACUC Meetings	The IACUC itself	Each meeting	Three years	Must include attendance, activities, and committee deliberations
Proposed activities and proposed significant changes (commonly called protocols and amendments)	The IACUC itself	Review each active proposal once yearly	Three years after the project is no longer active	Investigators must also be notified about the outcome of reviews of their proposals
Records of the semiannual reviews of programs of animal care and the semiannual inspection of the animal facility.	Institutional official	Twice yearly	Three years	Must include minority views, if any are submitted
Annual report of research facility	The USDA	Each December 1	Three years	Must include a description and justification of any IACUC-approved exceptions to the Animal Welfare Act. Must include a listing of the number of animals used, categorized by species and degree of invasiveness of the project
Report of suspension of any activity involving animals	Institutional official, who must in turn report the action to the USDA	Whenever an activity is suspended by the IACUC	Three years	Even a temporary suspension must be reported

Record	Recipient	Frequency	Retention	Comment
Disposition records for dogs and cats	The animal facility maintains and provides for inspectors when requested	Whenever an animal is added or removed from the facility's inventory	Three years after the animal is no longer held	These are usually maintained by the animal facility rather than the IACUC, but these important records are listed here for completeness
Medical records	Internal records kept by the animal facility or veterinary care unit	Whenever animals receive veterinary care	Many suggest keeping these records three years	These are usually maintained by the animal facility or the veterinary unit rather than the IACUC. There is no description of these records in USDA regulations; however, USDA inspectors hold that the existence of these records is implied by the general requirement for veterinary care

Note: All the records in the table must be made available to USDA Animal Welfare Inspectors on request.

are given in Tables 3.1 and 3.2. For each of these records, the minimal content and retention time is specified by law, regulation, or funding agency guidelines. We may add as much additional material to these records as we care to, and we may keep them for as much additional time as we deem necessary—but we must always comply with the minimum requirements.

If a proposed record is not mandated by an outside agency, and if the individual or unit suggesting the record will not be the one to maintain it, then do not implement it.

3.3   REGULATORY CREEP

Regulatory creep refers to the inescapable tendency for the interpretation of regulations to become more stringent over time, even in the absence of any change in the regulation itself. This happens whenever a conscientious person is charged with enforcing a rule. Whether the enforcer is a high school librarian, a university accountant, or an inspector for a regulatory agency, the conscientious regulator sees whatever flaws may exist in the rules as written and may seek to implement, by interpretation, requirements that were never written in the original rule. It is not unusual for an enforcing agency to request substantial new paperwork at a time when there has been no revision in the underlying rules or laws for decades.

Governmental agencies cannot arbitrarily require additional record keeping for regulated entities. Federal agencies are themselves regulated by the Administrative Procedure Act (5 USC Part 1, Chapter 5), which requires them to publish their proposed requirements in the *Federal Register* and consider public comment before implementing new regulatory requirements. If an agency has not gone through such a negotiated rulemaking process, it may suggest a new record, but is unlikely to be able to require it. If you find that a regulator is asking for a new record and you can find no requirement for the record in law or in the *Federal Register,* you should discuss the matter with the regulator's superior, your legislator, and perhaps your attorney.

3.4   COMMENTS ON CERTAIN MANDATED RECORDS

In this section, we will offer some of our own observations, opinions, and suggestions about a few of the most important mandated IACUC records.

3.4.1   PROTOCOLS

The word *protocol* refers to a short form summarizing the animal portions of a research project. The term does not occur in either the federal Animal Welfare Act regulations or the PHS Policy. Both the USDA and PHS require that the IACUC review procedures, activities, or proposals involving animals, but a special form for this purpose is not mentioned or required. It would be entirely possible for an IACUC at a very small facility to review the grant application directly without requiring an extra form, provided the grant gave an adequate description of the animal use in the project. IACUCs themselves invent protocols—forms that specifically address the animal issues of a project. There are as many different protocol forms as there are institutions. Regulators and IACUCs often have discussions about the specific contents of a particular institution's protocol form. Regulators may feel that a particular IACUC's form does not adequately address a particular issue and ask that it be revised. These discussions might best be resolved if the two agencies involved, the USDA and the Office for Protection from Research Risks (OPRR) designed a universal protocol form for use by all regulated institutions—but many people feel that this would be impractical.

Although the IACUC reviews protocols, it should not forget that it is actually giving its endorsement to the project as a whole—even to a grant application that the IACUC might not have seen. The IACUC should always have access to the complete proposal and be prepared to compare the contents of the protocol to the contents of the entire proposal.

Protocols often undergo extensive changes prior to approval, and they may be revised during a preview period prior to being distributed to the IACUC. Should the IACUC keep all the drafts and intermediate documents? Should the IACUC staff archive all the correspondence with the protocol? Personally, we would not keep copies of various draft versions of a protocol; multiple versions of the same document are redundant and cause confusion. After the final version of a protocol is approved by the IACUC, we mark it with a distinctive seal and destroy all earlier copies.

As an option, the IACUC may choose to keep all of its correspondence with investigators concerning their protocols. If there is correspondence back and forth, and the investigator is dealing with substantial issues of animal care and use, then we would choose to file such correspondence with the final protocol. If the correspondence is of a trivial nature, we would discard it. The goal should be to maximize the clarity and readability of the final file.

The USDA requires that protocols be reviewed annually, whereas the PHS requires that a new protocol be reviewed every three years. Many institutions resolve this inconsistency by performing a short or summary review of projects annually and requiring an entirely new protocol submission every three years.

3.4.2 MINUTES

Minutes describe the actions taken by the IACUC at convened meetings. Minutes may be verbose, including lengthy transcripts of discussions, or they may be brief and show only the final actions taken by the committee. Records that are verbose are laborious to maintain and might actually inhibit frank discussion. IACUC members may be reluctant to question a procedure or comment about a controversial issue if they feel their comments will be transcribed and distributed. On the other hand, records can be too brief. A set of minutes that recorded only votes but no discussion about a controversial issue might not help a subsequent IACUC understand why the decision was made.

The best minutes contain few, if any, comments about protocols that were approved as submitted. They do, however, contain concise summaries of conditions of approval, discussions of policy decisions, and summaries of inspection findings. Important correspondence relating to specific discussions should be attached to the minutes. In the interest of brevity, refer to the attachment in the minutes rather than trying to summarize or restate the contents of the attachment.

3.4.3 MINORITY REPORTS

Most IACUC decisions are made by compromise and consensus. The minutes, semiannual reviews, and other documents usually reflect the final consensus of the entire IACUC about an issue and do not attribute particular comments to particular individuals because the IACUC is speaking as a whole. When the IACUC speaks by consensus, all the members, in effect, have their signatures on the final document. This is not the case when minority reports are filed. Institutions are required to file minority reports when they are submitted with minutes, semiannual reviews, and annual reports to OPRR.

When the IACUC is divided in its opinion and a minority report is filed, then clarity requires that both the minority and majority reports be signed and filed. Any official document needs an author who will attest to its validity. When a minority report is filed, the author's signature proves the document's authenticity.

3.5 SEMIANNUAL INSPECTIONS/REVIEWS

Twice yearly, each IACUC must review the programs and facilities of the institution. Either two separate reports may be prepared, one for facilities inspections and one for programmatic issues, or the two documents may be combined into a single report.

Remember that the target audience of this report is the institutional official—generally a high level administrator. The semiannual report should be concise, readable, and convey information relevant to an administrator. It is to either tell the institutional official that everything is fine or to solicit the institutional official's help in improving the animal facilities or the policies of the institution.

3.6 AUTOMATING THE IACUC

Office automation can speed aspects of the review process and can reduce some of the drudgery involved in record keeping. Today, virtually all IACUCs make use of technology to the extent of providing their forms as word processing templates. Several companies market software products that at least partially automate the record keeping of the IACUC. Many other IACUCs develop their own systems. Whether you develop your own software or purchase a packaged product, consider the following points.

3.6.1 KEY CONCEPTS OF OFFICE AUTOMATION

3.6.1.1 IT WILL NOT BE CHEAP

Speed comes at a cost. It is not likely that office automation will either reduce the net cost of your IACUC or reduce the number of employees necessary to carry out its functions. Economies achieved in purely clerical tasks are often offset or exceeded by additional expenses of support staff, training, and software. The feasible goal should not be to reduce cost, but to improve service by reducing turnaround time through committee.

3.6.1.2 The True Record Is Still Paper

Have you ever known someone who lost an important document because a floppy disk failed or his computer's hard disk burned out? It is a common and gut-wrenching experience. Most magnetic media are stable for a few years at best. On the other hand, there are many written documents (the Book of Kells, original Guttenberg Bibles, and the Declaration of Independence, to name a few) that are hundreds of years old, still here, and still legible.

Electronic documents are easily edited but are also easily falsified. Although it is possible to create electronic signatures, the present state of technology provides no seal of authenticity as simple and elegant as a signature.

Electronic communications can help us prepare written documents more accurately and efficiently, but our opinion is that the end product should still be a paper document with a signature.

3.6.1.3 Simple Solutions Are More Likely to Succeed

The last decade has seen numerous catastrophic failures to implement propriety, large-scale computer systems in governmental agencies and in the private sector. (Particularly well-known examples would include large-scale boondoggles at the federal Internal Review Service and California's State Automated Welfare System.) The same period has seen an amazingly successful growth of two relatively simple Internet-related technologies: e-mail and the World Wide Web. As many as twenty million ordinary Americans are able to send each other e-mail and order everything from books to flower seeds over the World Wide Web. It is the relative simplicity and openness of these two technologies that have made them successful. The key is not high tech but appropriate tech.

3.6.2 TOOLS OF THE INTERNET

The components of technology most likely to be cost effective in the hands of the IACUC are simple ones such as e-mail and the World Wide Web.

3.6.2.1 E-Mail

E-mail allows people to communicate out of sequence with each other. It combines the depth and precision of written correspondence with the ability of an answering machine to take messages and replay them at the recipient's convenience. Unlike any other means of correspondence, it allows contents of conversations to be edited, pasted into other documents, redistributed, and even printed. A single worker can handle many more contacts in a day via e-mail than he or she can via the telephone or land mail.

3.6.2.2 The World Wide Web

The World Wide Web provides an economical way of publishing documents. Operating a web server on your computer allows you to make an infinite number of copies of any document you choose and distribute the document to anyone in the world who is willing to receive it. Place your blank protocols on the Web, and you will no longer have to answer the telephone, make copies, stuff envelopes, or pay for postage. The Web allows computers of different types to share documents easily. Documents placed on the Web are equally readable by users of Apple, Microsoft, and Unix-based computers.

Using e-mail and the Web, a faculty member can decide at midnight he or she needs a blank form, fill it out at 1:00 a.m. and send the completed form back to you as an e-mail attachment. You arrive at your office at 8:00 a.m. the next morning, and the completed form is in your computer without your having to spend any time with the investigator at all. The investigator could have done this from a different building or a different state with equal ease.

3.6.2.3 The Pre-Cambrian Period

The evolution of technology at the University of California, Davis, has followed a path taking us up from Olduvai Gorge to the dawn of a new millennium. Our IACUC has been using computers in some capacity for the past 15 years. During this time, we have witnessed many successes as well as failures in our evolutionary experiments.

We began reviewing protocols in 1984, just one year before IACUCs were mandated to do so by federal law. The protocols were first held in three cardboard magazine boxes on my desk labeled "Incoming Protocols," "Protocols to Committee," and "Protocols to File." Protocols in other categories, such as "Approved Pending Clarification," were stacked in piles marked with yellow sticky notes. The IACUC received 683 protocols to review that year. When the first few boxes were bursting at the seams and when the desk became so cluttered that the top was no longer visible under piles of documents, it became obvious that we needed to organize the protocols differently. The first step was to file all the protocols sequentially and then maintain information about the status of each protocol in a database.

3.6.2.3.1   Stratum one: the database

IACUCs with a large volume of protocols need to track their activities. A minimal database will not contain the text of each protocol, but will record the name of the investigator, the species, the project title, the important dates, and other information you will likely need at some future time. Using any popular, off-the-shelf database program, your IACUC should be able to generate lists of protocols to be placed on the agenda of upcoming meetings. This program can also be used to remind principal investigators, or PIs, to submit their protocols for annual reviews to send letters to funding bodies verifying approval, to print lists of investigators authorized to purchase certain numbers of certain species, and to help prepare a variety of other useful reports.

In 1985, we began managing our protocols with an in-house database program written in DbaseIII + , which went through a few iterations of added functions over the next few years. It was eventually translated into another computer language called CA-Clipper. On the whole, it has been successful, but it lacks many of the refinements now expected in consumer software. In 1998, we complain about it daily, and hope to retire it soon, but we are still using it.

3.6.2.3.2   Stratum two: the inspection database—adaptive
radiation followed by extinction

After some initial success with a program to track protocols, we attempted to digitize and automate the IACUC inspections of our animal facilities. The animal facilities at UC Davis comprise over 1500 rooms in 226 different buildings. There are twenty vivaria or "management units," each of whose programs receives a separate semiannual review.

In the mid-1980s, our inspection reports tended to consist largely of lists of minor physical facility deficiencies. An important function of our inspections was to prioritize maintenance requests for our physical plant. Our thinking was that by organizing our reports into coded lists of deficiencies and locations, we would be able to create summaries that would help with management decisions. ("We have 130 rooms in which there are small cracks in the plaster; let's group them by building and create a work crew to go out and fix them all in one week.")

Our experiments with computerized inspections ultimately did not fit our needs. Our computer-generated reports had several failings:

1. Recording long lists of deficiencies, however minor, gave a negative tone to the reports, which tended to discourage, rather than inspire, the animal-care staff
2. Programmatic issues did not lend themselves to a check-off list—they required an insightful and diplomatic discussion with the management of the facility
3. The intended audience of the semiannual review is the management of the facility and the institutional official.

The report needs to be concise, readable, and comprehensible to others in future years. A list is just a list, however accurate its contents.

After a number of experiments with other inspection formats, our semiannual reviews evolved into an entirely text-based format. We hope our inspection will consist of a thoughtful and literate evaluation of the facility and its management. We use the Association for Assessment and Accreditation of Laboratory Animal Care's letters of evaluation as our model to the greatest extent possible. Deficiencies are discussed in a broad way, with examples given. We do not attempt to catalog every single fault we may have noted in the facility. When appropriate, we also point out the positive, noting the strengths of the facility and its staff. Each report is short, often no longer than a few pages, and the emphasis is on the positive actions a facility should take to better its program.

The consensus seems to be that the animal-care staff prefers a text format over all our attempts to digitize the process. We may automate this process to the extent of scheduling inspections but not to the extent of digitizing the reports themselves.

3.6.2.3.3   Stratum three: throwing away the typewriter

In 1984, our standard practice was to distribute paper copies of the blank animal protocol that were then filled in by typewriter. The form was not produced in-house, but was actually typeset by a professional printer. Not until about 1990 were computers cheap enough and software simple enough to allow ordinary users to design forms easily.

By the early 1990s, blank protocol forms were generated in-house with personal computers rather than being sent to a printer, and the dominant means of distribution had become word-processing templates on disk. Distributing blanks on disk made it easier for the investigators to create and edit their documents, but this was actually more work for the IACUC staff. It takes longer and is more costly to copy a floppy disk than to copy a paper form.

3.6.2.3.4   Stratum four: webbed feat

The IACUCs often find it necessary to distribute information to faculty and animal-care staff. Instructions for completing protocols, IACUC policies on a variety of issues, announcements, tables of drug doses, and other information is commonly sent to a large number of people. OPRR specifically requests that each institution's

Animal Welfare Assurance be made available to the faculty. This is a lengthy document; hence, thoughts about mailing it to over 1000 principal investigators were somewhat daunting.

In the late 1980s, we began publishing a small newsletter to keep our staff and faculty up to date. This involved printing over 1500 copies of a multipage newsletter and mailing it to the appropriate audience. Today we just use our web server and e-mail to deliver the same information to the same audience. Permanent documents and references are published on our web server rather than on paper, and announcements and news items are distributed to supervisory animal-care staff using an e-mail list server.

3.6.2.3.5   Stratum five: the electronic carrier pigeon

With the explosion in popularity of the Internet after 1995, both the hardware and skills necessary to exchange documents electronically became widely available. By early 1997, we had stopped receiving requests for blank protocols on disk. As this chapter is written in May 1998, 96 percent of the employees of UC Davis, as well as the entire faculty, have an e-mail address. Investigators are now able to download current versions of blank protocols directly from the IACUC's web site onto their own computer. Typewritten documents have become so rare as to merit a comment when they arrive, and it is virtually unheard of to request paper blanks. But even more significant than the ability to distribute the blanks is our ability to edit the documents we receive.

As any IACUC staffer knows, most if not all protocols must be revised many times as they work their way through the approval process. If the document received by the IACUC is paper, then only the PI can edit the original document. Even a minor change in the language of the protocol, such as an addition to the literature search, requires sending the protocol back to the PI to be edited on the PI's computer. Editing the protocol directly in the IACUC office can save several days' turnaround time.

With the widespread adoption of e-mail by our institution, electronic submission of protocol documents is becoming common, although still not the universal way of submitting a protocol. Presently this is usually done by sending the binary word processed protocol as an attachment to e-mail.

We presently receive approximately 30 percent of protocols as attachments to e-mail messages. Opening the e-mail places the intact word processing document on the recipient's hard disk in fully editable form. This offers several advantages, but those advantages come at a cost.

When the protocol is received as an attachment, one avoids the delay associated with land mail, and the document can be directly edited in the IACUC office. Turnaround time is reduced. However, IACUC staff time associated with editing and computer support tasks has increased. Computer users on our campus are not confined to a single software or hardware platform. The newly arrived protocol may have been prepared on a Macintosh or a Microsoft/Intel-based PC, and it may have been edited with a variety of word processing programs. Users also vary widely in their computer skills; they will occasionally make changes to the protocol blank that significantly complicates further editing. Also, a surprising high percentage of documents we receive as attachments have been contaminated with trojans or viruses.

To date, the widespread submission of protocols by e-mail has involved the IACUC staff in:

1. Translating incoming protocols from one word processing format to another.
2. Reinstalling fonts and formatting what may have been damaged by the user.
3. Protecting their own computers from daily assault by trojans and viruses.

These computer support activities demand training and time on our part—something not necessary in the past.

Submission of protocols via e-mail has been a mixed blessing. We find that when the PI is skilled in the use of his or her computer, the savings in time to the PI and to the IACUC staff is considerable. When the PI is relatively unskilled in the use of the computer, we find that the IACUC staff become trainers, not only with respect to animal care issues, but with respect to computer skills and information technology. In addition to teaching PIs how to restrain a furry mouse, we find ourselves teaching them over the telephone about the intricacies of downloading with the one-button vs. the two-button mouse.

We are currently seeking a way to receive and edit protocols electronically without having to support numerous word processing formats. We believe that the solution will be to move all electronic submissions to the World Wide Web. It would be possible to allow protocols to be completed via a web page using a Web browser rather than a word processing program. We feel this is the wave of the future, but we have not implemented such a program at this time.

3.6.2.3.6   *Stratum six: virtual meetings*

The members of the IACUC can also use e-mail to converse with each other. At our campus, the IACUC maintains two electronic mailing lists, one for IACUC members and another for supervisory animal-care staff. The latter is used primarily for announcements of classes and other informational items aimed at the animal-care staff.

The IACUC's own e-mail list is often used to discuss protocols prior to a convened meeting. Printed copies of all the protocols on each agenda are mailed to IACUC members prior to the meeting. IACUC members are asked to read each protocol critically and, should they have any questions or concerns about a particular protocol, they are asked to forward their questions to the IACUC staff. The staff members collect and summarize the questions associated with each protocol and e-mail the assembled questions to the PI. The PI's response is then e-mailed back to the staff member, with the result that all questions can usually be answered before the meeting. Our goal is to produce a protocol that is perfect and complete by the day of the meeting, so that no protocols have to be held or tabled for further information at the meeting.

Should additional points or comments be raised at the meeting, the IACUC often gives "approval pending clarification" at the meeting. This allows the IACUC staff to gather the requested information from the PI, distribute the additional information to the IACUC via the mailing list, and then issue final approval (as a designated reviewer) should no further concerns be brought forward.

3.6.2.3.6.1   The possibilities and limits of virtual meetings—Many actions of the IACUC can take place only at a convened, physical meeting. Examples are those actions requiring a vote of the assembled group, such as acceptance of the semiannual reviews, approval of the minutes of the last meeting, or suspension of an ongoing activity. The approval of protocols, however, does not require a vote of the entire IACUC and does not need to take place at a convened meeting. OPRR policy and USDA regulations allow delegation of the approval of protocols to a single member of the IACUC, provided that each member of the IACUC has been given a list of all the projects to be acted upon. It would be possible to design procedures under which the approval of protocols would be technically delegated to a single reviewer, but only after an e-mail discussion in which the entire IACUC participated. It would even be possible to conduct the discussion using a World Wide Web based conferencing system. The only caveat would have to be that if any single member of the IACUC wished to discuss a particular protocol at a convened meeting with a quorum, then that particular protocol would have to be held for the convened face-to-face meeting and could not be delegated to the designated reviewer.

Although approval of most protocols via "meetings on the web" is a possibility, it is not something we have ever chosen to implement at our facility. At this point, our use of e-mail to act on protocols has been limited to actions taking place after a convened meeting rather than preceding it. The general pattern has been that a protocol has been discussed, and while there are no major concerns, there are sufficient unresolved details that the protocol cannot be approved as presented at the time of the meeting. At the meeting, the IACUC delegates approval to a single member pending completion of a task (such as the PI's staff attending a class) or written clarification of some aspect of the project. After the designated member verifies that the IACUC's requirements have been fulfilled, the member informs the IACUC and approves the protocol.

3.6.2.3.7   Stratum seven: tracking numbers—talking
*   to the other guys*

It has become a regulatory expectation that institutions should be able to associate animal purchases with particular protocols. If the IACUC has approved a project for 50 mice, it should be impossible for the investigator to order a higher number of mice without the prior consent of the IACUC. Since the IACUC and the purchasing entity for the institution are separate entities, they will need to establish a mechanism for the IACUC to authorize the purchase of animals for a particular PI.

At our institution, this is currently done by providing Purchasing with a paper "List of Approved Projects," which Purchasing consults prior to placing an order. Increasingly, it is a regulatory expectation that there be an active system under which the IACUC can monitor the purchasing process day by day, and in which each animal purchased is subtracted from the number the PI is allowed to purchase. This is easy to implement at small institutions with centralized ordering, but more difficult at large institutions where ordering is decentralized.

Several companies sell software packages that automate many aspects of vivarium management. These packages are worth investigating, especially if your vivarium and your IACUC are tightly integrated and flexible enough to mold their own operations to the software. These packages are more difficult to use in large institutions where the vivarium must interact with other accounting systems on the campus.

Many institutions find it necessary to create their own software to manage the vivarium, control animal ordering, and share purchasing data with the IACUC. Developing such software is always difficult; it generally means that the vivarium must hire a full-time programmer. At UC Davis and at many other institutions, the automatic integration of the IACUC's data with the purchasing process remains a distant goal.

3.6.2.3.8   Stratum eight: daylight at the surface: privacy and public access

A private corporation or private university will generally choose to keep all IACUC communications private. This does not necessarily rule out using the Internet as a vehicle for exchanging documents, but it calls for additional effort and the recruitment of a highly skilled information technology staff. A corporation may also implement Internet technologies within an "intranet," which uses all the same tools but lacks any physical connection to computers outside the corporate walls.

Public institutions are often required to make most, if not all, of their documents available to the public on request. The particulars, such as exactly what is a public document, vary from state to state, but, in general, IACUCs at public institutions should plan that most or all of their records will be available to the public.

In California, unlike many other states, University of California IACUC meetings can be closed meetings—only the members of the IACUC and others of their choosing can attend. This is a blessing to the IACUC, because it allows an informality and frankness in discussion that might be lost if members were afraid their every comment might be broadcast out of context. The records of the IACUC are, however, public, with certain exceptions. These exceptions are:

1. Under California's Information Practices Act, the names, addresses, and home phone numbers of state employees may not be released. Because the protocol often contains this information for emergency purposes, this information must be redacted before the document can be released.

2. The Federal Animal Welfare Act gives protection to "trade secrets" and other proprietary information. In our experience, it has been extremely uncommon for animal protocols to contain detailed proprietary information that could be withheld under this provision. If a protocol did contain such information, that portion should be deleted if the protocol is to be made public. An argument could also be made that an unfunded grant

proposal, rather like a manuscript in progress, contains proprietary ideas which require withholding unfunded protocols from public access. This argument could be used to justify withholding a protocol only until such time as it had been funded.

3. A public record is defined as a record that the agency keeps in the course of ordinary business. Certainly the statutory records shown in Tables 3.1 and 3.2 would be public records in California, because they must be kept in the course of ordinary business. Are early drafts of protocols, notes to investigators, and the e-mails of IACUC members public? The answer is that they are public records if they are kept in the course of ordinary business. If they are routinely discarded, then they are not public records. The IACUC should therefore carefully consider what it chooses to archive and what it chooses to discard. In general, it is best to establish policies about what is kept and what is not, and then follow those policies scrupulously. At UC Davis, we file all relevant documents and correspondence pertaining to a protocol as a paper copy with the final protocol. If an electronic document contains important information about a protocol, we print it and archive it with the paper file. We do not routinely keep old e-mails or archive the correspondence on our list servers.

3.7   PUBLIC RECORDS

Responding to a request for a public record can be a costly process. A very general or sweeping public records act request can require an inordinate amount of labor to complete, and the IACUC would be prohibited by law from imposing charges for anything other than the direct cost of making copies. Increasingly, public agencies are making the public portions of their public documents available on the World Wide Web. There are many examples of this within the federal government, the most recent being the USDA's recent decision to place its inspections of animal research facilities on a searchable Web page. This can potentially save the agency and the public entity a great deal of money. If public records are available on the World Wide Web and visible in any public library, it is entirely reasonable for the public agency to deny all other requests for copies of the documents and simply refer them to the Web site.

Placing public documents on the Web is a win—win situation for both the public entity and the individual seeking access to the record. The requester gets the document more easily and quickly, and the public agency is spared the labor associated with searching, unfiling, copying, refiling and mailing the record.

Investigators are much less likely to be comfortable with their records being placed on the Web. To them, I would simply point out that their protocol is a public document whether or not it is available via the Web. A request for the record will be granted in either case; it is simply less costly to fill the request if the document is on the Web. Federally funded research proposals, including all the financial information, are probably already available on the World Wide Web at the funding agency's web site.

While some investigators might prefer anonymity, there is some public relations benefit to providing full and accurate information about a project to the general public. Opponents of research have often distorted the contents of protocols beyond recognition in their attempts to slander a particular project. It might be easier to defend a project and dismiss the distortions if the original is readily available to the press and the general public. See Section 4.15.

At the UC Davis, our ideal system for managing protocols would be based on the technologies of the Internet. Correspondence with investigators would be mostly electronic, and the protocols themselves would be Web-based and would be completed using a browser. Those aspects of protocols and other documents that by law ought to be available to the public would be available to the general public using the World Wide Web. The deliberations of the IACUC would be confidential, but their decisions would be public. The purchasing of animals, the operation of the vivarium, the cost accounting of grants, and the documentation of training would be integrated databases that would be available in real time on the desktops of everyone who had a legitimate need for the data.

We are not there yet, but we shall try to make our work as efficient, direct, and open as we possibly can. Technology will play a role in this process, but, we hope, not at the expense of human interaction and direct involvement with the animals in our care.

SOURCES AND SUGGESTED READING

Code of Federal Regulations: Regulations in support of the federal Animal Welfare Act, 9 CFR Subpart A Section 2.35 and 2.31.

United States Public Health Service Animal Welfare Policy (PHS Policy), Sections IV.E. and IV.F.

Garnett N. and Potkay, S., Use of electronic communications for IACUC functions, *ILAR J.*, 37(4), 190–192. 1995.

Freedom of Information Act, and amendments, 1996, Title 5, U.S. Code Part 1, Chapter 5(II), Section 522.

California Public Records Act, California Government Code, Sections 6250–6265.

The Information Practices Act of 1977, California Civil Code, Sections 1798.1–1798.78.

The Administrative Procedure Act, 5 U.S. Code, Part 1, Chapter 5.

4 IACUC Issues in Academia

Stephen P. Schiffer, D.V.M., M.S.

CONTENTS

4.1   INTRODUCTION

Although few issues are exclusively the province of academia, there are many situations that tend to arise more often in a college or university than in industry. This chapter will address issues that generally confront IACUCs in academic institutions.

4.2   THE ROLE OF THE IACUC

Academic institutions are responsible for ensuring that the use of animals in research, education, and testing (if applicable) conforms to acceptable ethical, humane, and scientific standards. A strong regulatory emphasis is placed on in-house senior management to provide oversight responsibility for animal care and use programs, which, in turn, depends upon the triumvirate of the institutional official (IO), the attending veterinarian (AV), and the IACUC for implementation. The IO, usually the institution's president or CEO, is the individual to whom the institution has given the authority and responsibility to enforce and supervise the requirements of AWA and PHS policy.[1, 2] While each of these units has its own function and jurisdiction, their interrelationships are critical to the overall operation of the program and help set the tone within the institution. The strength of the animal care program in academia will reflect the relationship of the IACUC with the IO, the AV, and the research faculty it oversees.

The relationship between the IO and the IACUC may not be obvious on a day-to-day basis, yet it provides the philosophic foundation for much of what the IACUC does. In large universities, the IO function may be delegated to a high-ranking administrator with oversight responsibilities for the research program, like the dean of research.[3] Beyond the primary role of administering the animal program and promoting open communication with the medical school, veterinary school, and other units of the institution involved in animal care and use, the IO should rely upon the IACUC to maintain exemplary animal care and facilities and to support and promote research in compliance with existing standards.[4] By doing so, the IO establishes the institutional climate and provides the commitment to animal care through the IACUC. This can be measured in several ways. Financial support, personnel, and facility infrastructure are the most obvious. Achieving and maintaining AAALAC accreditation is a strong indicator of an IO's commitment. AAALAC accreditation assures the scientific and lay communities that laboratory animals will be used humanely, that humans will be protected from animal and research related hazards, that variables that could affect research results are minimized, and that there is compliance with all applicable laws. Another important measure of the IO's commitment is seen in the way the IACUC is supported, especially when it tries to enforce institutional policies and legal requirements. Strong support by the IO when the IACUC faces difficult situations will affirm the authority and stature of the IACUC within the institution. Conversely, the IACUC's role is undermined if the IO does not have the power and authority, or willingness, to deal with schools, departments, or faculty that resist being part of the program. For the good of the institution, the IO must be knowledgeable, available, and have a vested interest in the success of the animal care program, particularly on behalf of the science and teaching disciplines.

The relationship between the IACUC and the AV is rather complex. The AV is almost always a member of the IACUC, yet it is part of the IACUC's job to oversee the AV's operation. This gives rise to the question, should the AV serve as the IACUC Chairperson?[5] In smaller academic programs, the physical location and administrative personnel for the IACUC and AV offices may be the same; investigators may confuse the two and consider them as one administrative entity. It is important that everyone knows that there is a separation of powers between the IACUC and the AV—somewhat analogous to the legislative and executive branches of government. Faculty may believe that the IACUC's decisions and policies are made by the AV when in fact the AV is just one member of the committee. Another consequence of integrated offices is that it becomes easy to place the burden of conducting most of the time-consuming and thankless tasks of the IACUC on the AV or the AV's staff members. The AV should function as an individual member of the IACUC who supplies special expertise in relevant areas. The AV should not be the sole regulator.

One challenge that IACUCs in academia must face is the perceived administrative burden placed upon the faculty. Investigators claim they spend 10 to 20 percent of their time doing administrative tasks mandated by the federal government's growing "appetite for red tape."[6] As a result, some faculty members may exhibit resistance to the IACUC on the premise that it is nothing but another part of the bureaucracy (see Figure 4.1).

The IACUC should strive to maintain and promote an open and cooperative relationship with the faculty,[4] but, not uncommonly, it has to deal with the "prima donna syndrome." This sector needs repeated reminding of the importance of compliance and the consequences of noncompliance with the law. How an IACUC deals with such individuals or departments will depend upon the particular situation at a particular time. A sage professor serving as the IACUC chair for a major academic institution once characterized the IACUC's role and relationship with the faculty as a paternalistic one—requiring patience and a firm hand.

4.3   IACUC MEMBERSHIP

Both the AWA and the PHS policy are clear, although discrepant, in their requirements for IACUC composition. They establish the minimum membership and permit an institution to have as many members as they want, providing no more than three people come from any one institutional unit (e.g., department). While the CEO/IO is the one who appoints the members, the IACUC chair should be consulted about appointments to ensure that the committee has an effective membership. In an academic institution, beyond those members mandated by law such as the community representative, certain review criteria may be used to achieve a balanced membership. First, each major entity such as a department or college that conducts animal research should have representation. Some of these may have standing slots on the committee, such as a college of agriculture. Second, there should be balanced representation of the faculty who use different types of animals: rodents, large animals, primates, or wildlife. Third, there should be balanced representation of scientists from the major research disciplines such as basic science, applied science, neuroscience, cancer, pharmaceuticals, and cardiovascular–renal–pulmonary research. More than one researcher from these programs may be helpful; it allows for the protocol review burden to be shared. Having practicing scientists on the committee has two advantages. It gives the IACUC a greater sense of peer-review status, which may make it less likely to be considered adversarial. Additionally, well-trained scientists can provide a critical evaluation of protocols from a scientific method perspective.

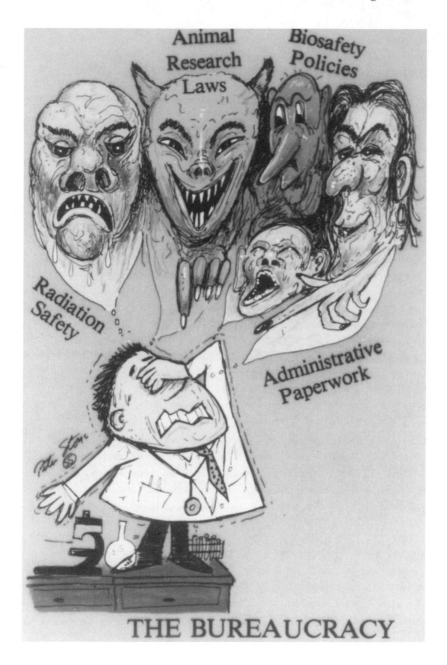

See Section 4.9 on Scientific Merit. The final criterion is to have certain specialists on the committee, such as surgeons, anesthesiologists, and bioethicists. Drawing upon the bank of experts in the institution can be very beneficial to the IACUC. Small institutions that have limited resources in personnel may consider implementing consortium-type arrangements with nearby organizations in order to attract enough qualified and interested individuals to their IACUC.[7]

4.4   INTERACTIVENESS OF THE IACUC

In an academic research center, where animal care protocols may involve a wide range of species and subject areas, IACUCs must, in addition to observing the mandates of AWA, take into consideration the U.S. government principles for the utilization and care of vertebrate animals used in testing, research, and training.

Outside experts may be consulted for particularly complex protocols. In certain situations, however, the IACUC may not feel comfortable approving a protocol as submitted. In these situations, the IACUC can become rather interactive with the research project if it chooses to do so. For example, IACUC members may ask to witness or even experience, the first set of experiments performed on the animals. This may or may not be reassuring to members who question the procedure. For protocols which are truly novel—where there is no data or prior experience—and which may involve significant morbidity or mortality, the IACUC may ask the investigator to perform a pilot study first[8] and report back to the committee concerning end-point modifiers. Although a researcher may consider these actions intrusive, it is essential that the IACUC feels comfortable with what is being approved.

4.5   SIZE AND DIVERSITY OF THE
RESEARCH PROGRAM

The size of the academic institution has a direct relationship to the size and diversity of the animal research programs that the IACUC must oversee. This impacts the IACUC in several ways. First, the larger the institution, the greater the number of academic jurisdictions (e.g., departments, colleges), and the greater the number of animal facilities. While a centralized animal facility is ideal from a practical perspective, this may not be practical for a large campus. Therefore, IACUC facility inspections need to be coordinated to cover all regulated areas, including those off-site, in a timely manner. Second, as the institutional size increases, so does the work load for the IACUC. For example, IACUCs for small institutions may review fewer than 5 protocols in a year, whereas in large universities this may amount to 700 protocols. Having an adequate number of members with expertise on the committee can ensure that no one person has to carry an undue burden of protocol review and that protocols will be reviewed on time. Third, as the institutional size increases, so does the variety of animal-use projects. A single institution may have animal care programs in support of professional medical and veterinary schools, agricultural research, and wildlife/biology projects. This has become problematic for IACUCs since the AWA, the PHS policy, and the *Guide for the Care and Use of Laboratory Animals* were designed primarily with biomedical research in mind.[1, 2, 8] As a result, these provisions may not be suitable for the special conditions required for the scientific investigations of farm animals and wild vertebrate animals.[3, 8, 9] For example, at land-grant universities where the majority of university-related food and fiber research and teaching in such areas as dairy science and poultry science is conducted, there can be a major difference between the animal-care practices that support biomedical research as compared to agricultural research.[10] Agricultural animal research most often is conducted under conditions representative of agricultural practices. The IACUC needs to distinguish between biomedical and agricultural uses of farm animals.[8, 11] To properly monitor the use of farm animals in agricultural research and teaching, IACUCs need to use criteria such as those outlined in the *Guide for the Care and Use of Agricultural Animals in Agricultural Research and Teaching*.[12] Similarly, many academic institutions have research and teaching programs that involve fish, amphibians, reptiles, birds, and various wild mammals. Application of rigorous PHS policies to wild animals may be difficult because there is no single set of guidelines. Although it is the responsibility of the IACUC to ensure that wildlife research is humane, it may be dealing with a species about which there may be scant information. This difficulty can be resolved when the IACUC, veterinarians, and wildlife experts work together.[13]

Protocols involving wild animals may be further complicated because they involve field investigations. While ensuring that local, state, and federal regulations are observed, there are a variety of guidelines available for conducting such work with fish,[14] amphibians and reptiles,[15] wild birds,[16] and wild mammals.[17] If the composition of the IACUC is well-balanced, then most of these protocol situations are manageable. However, some institutions have created two or more IACUCs—one for biomedical research and another for agricultural and wildlife animal studies. If an institution chooses to have multiple IACUCs, then the challenge is to ensure uniformity in implementing IACUC oversight activities. Regardless of how the challenge is addressed by the IACUCs, the basic principles of humane care and ethical standards still apply for all species.

Finally, it is the IACUC's responsibility to make sure that individuals who conduct procedures on animals are properly trained and qualified. This can be a real challenge for a large academic institution because animal research personnel includes faculty, postdoctoral, graduate, undergraduate, summer students, research technicians, and visitors who may be collaborators. Further, there can be a frequent turnover of these individuals. Because there are currently few programs for certifying the competence of investigators or research technicians in the conduct of animal procedures, IACUCs must establish in-house criteria by which investigators are judged.[7] Other than the subject matter mandated by the AWA, the content of all training programs should be tailored to the internal needs of the institution to ensure relevancy for the participants. Tracking and documenting an individual's participation in the training program before that person begins actual work with the animals can also pose problems. This challenge can be met if there is some form of controlled access, such as a computer card system, to the animal facility.

4.6   FUNDING SOURCES AND DEADLINES

IACUCs must review and approve all animal usage before an investigator can conduct any project using live vertebrate animals for research, teaching, or testing. There are, however, no mandated time frames for completing this review process. Because most research at academic institutions is funded by extramural agencies or sources as part of the peer review process, these extramural granting agencies usually have their own timelines for requiring IACUC approval of a proposed animal study. This means that the agency must receive documentation of IACUC review and approval; otherwise, the grant proposal will not be considered. As a result, an occasional situation arises in which a faculty member finds a grant proposal held up and threatened with being discarded from review simply because of inadequate IACUC documentation. These situations are stressful and sometimes require heroic efforts to obtain appropriate review, approval, and submitted documentation without compromising IACUC principles. To avoid this kind of situation, three things are important. First, the rules for IACUC review and approval, and an approximate turnaround time, should be clearly outlined for every faculty member who intends to use animals. Second, deadlines for protocol submission and meeting frequencies should be clearly outlined. Investigators must know about the specific requirements for animal studies to be funded by that particular agency—the National Institutes of Health (NIH) and the National Science Foundation (NSF) normally allow 60 days for approval after the deadline submission date; the American Heart Association (AHA) requires that studies which propose to use animals must be reviewed and approved by the IACUC before the grant is submitted for peer review.

Finally, it may be advisable for the IACUC, with input from the IO, to develop a policy for dealing with the investigator who repeatedly puts grants in jeopardy because of failure to work within the system. Late protocol submissions or poorly written protocols invite rejections.

4.7   REQUIREMENTS FOR PROTOCOL REVIEW

Not all animal research is regulated. For example, privately funded biomedical studies on rats and mice are not regulated. Some animal activities in academic institutions with agricultural, veterinary, and wildlife programs also remain unregulated. Specifically, those activities or projects that are not funded by the PHS or a governmental agency and do not involve AWA regulated species technically are not required to have an IACUC-approved protocol. Some institutions may have small colonies of ectothermic, cold-blooded vertebrates supported by nonfederal dollars. Others have teaching laboratories that use animal organs obtained from slaughterhouses. Still others have live animal displays (e.g., snakes in a biology department) or on-site rodeos or fish kept in aquaria in the workplace, or even campus pest programs involving vertebrate species, feral cats, rodents, birds, and wildlife.[18, 19] While some of these activities are regulated by other rules, they are not covered by the more standard biomedical regulations or funding agencies. The decision to require any or all of these activities to be reviewed and approved by the IACUC rests with each institution. Some institutions may choose to review them, while others will not.

The major document that provides guidance on this issue is the institution's OPRR Letter of Assurance (LOA). This federally approved document specifically indicates the extent to which that institution's LOA is to apply. Some institutions elect to apply the document to all animals, while others elect to apply it only to the PHS-funded projects. There are advantages and disadvantages to either choice. If there is a decision to restrict the application of the LOA, only those entities listed in the document will be entitled to use the assurance number for grant and contract submissions to PHS agencies. Further, the institution will need to document that the animal care and use program funded by a non-PHS source is entirely separate and distinct, physically and programmatically, from PHS-supported activities before the OPRR will consider its exclusion from the institutional assurance. Unless there is such total separation, OPRR cannot accept the potential risks presented to the animals involved in the PHS-funded research.[20] Institutions should also keep in mind the public perception that institutions not wishing to conduct portions of their animal research or teaching in accordance with policy may be applying a double standard of animal care to the detriment of overall animal health and well-being. For this reason, the LOA usually applies to all of the institution's animal research, teaching, and testing without restriction, based upon the source of funding.

4.8   WHO CAN SERVE AS PRINCIPAL INVESTIGATOR ON A PROTOCOL?

In an academic setting, there are many situations in which someone or some group other than a faculty member has the main responsibility for an animal project. For example, graduate students and postdoctoral trainees often have their own animal research projects. Another example is a private company that wants to conduct a teaching laboratory for health care professionals to demonstrate a new technology. The issue for the IACUC is who can serve as the principal investigator (PI) on the animal protocol? There is little regulatory guidance on this issue; the decision rests with the institution. On the surface, this may not seem to be a major dilemma, but if the animal protocol is to be considered a written contract between the animal user and the institution, then accountability becomes a key issue, particularly if something were to go wrong with the project (e.g., evidence of gross noncompliance). A straightforward strategy that an IACUC can use is to require that the PI on the protocol be a member of the faculty. This clearly places responsibility with an accountable individual. The one exception to this might be if a student or postdoctoral fellow is submitting an individual, outside grant proposal. If a nonfaculty individual is allowed to serve as the PI on a protocol, then faculty sponsorship and signatures are essential. Ultimate responsibility resides with that faculty member. Whatever strategy is used, the IACUC should have a clear, written policy on who can serve as the PI on an animal protocol.

4.9   SCIENTIFIC MERIT

A contentious issue within the academic community concerns scientific merit review.[21] Who has the responsibility for ensuring that animal research has an acceptable level of scientific merit? Is it the investigator, the institution, the IACUC, or the funding agency? Since many, if not most, protocols are subjected to extensive external scientific review as part of the funding process, the IACUC can be relatively assured of appropriate scientific review. However, the IACUC cannot totally avoid the issue of scientific merit. External funding reviews should be viewed as additional assurance, rather than the only assurance, that the research has value. While not an expert in every field, a properly constituted IACUC with broad-based expertise can perform a valid evaluation of scientific merit by asking investigators the appropriate questions and by assessing how well an experiment is constructed. Since humane animal use implies morally appropriate animal use, IACUCs must determine that the procedures before them are expertly planned and necessary.[22] **It is inhumane to use animals for bad science.** Having trained biomedical scientists with an understanding of scientific methodology should be in the IACUC's purview; the IACUC can judge the merit of a protocol at this fundamental level. Expertise in the precise area of the research is not always necessary. Very simply, a good scientist hates bad science. Scientists on an IACUC sometimes are the strongest critics of poorly designed animal research protocols.

The question then arises, what should the IACUC do when dealing with animal studies that will not undergo outside review for scientific merit? Many IACUCs require sign-off by the investigator's department chairman or an internal review committee. This makes signers responsible for providing assurance that the proposed studies have been designed and will be performed with due consideration of their relevance to human or animal health, the advancement of knowledge, or the good of society. With guidance from the IO, each IACUC should develop guidelines for dealing with situations where the merit of the project is in question.

4.10   THE USE OF HAZARDOUS AGENTS

As the overseer of the animal care and use program for an institution, the IACUC has broad responsibilities that can include identifying the occupational health and safety concerns for those who work with animals. While this covers many issues beyond the scope of this chapter, the IACUC protocol can ask if there will be any use of hazardous agents (i.e., biological, chemical, physical, and radioactive) or public health concerns (e.g., taking an animal to a human hospital for magnetic resonance imaging).[23] The challenge is to link review and approval of the animal work by the IACUC with the review and approval by the appropriate safety committee (e.g., biosafety or hospital infection control).

4.11   USE OF ANIMALS FOR TEACHING

Academic institutions with educational programs involving the life sciences also entail the use of animals. Animals may be used for a wide range of instructional purposes—for undergraduate college students, professional veterinary, medical, or nursing students, practicing physicians and surgeons—to teach anatomy, surgery, and to demonstrate the newest technologies. Because this kind of teaching comes under the purview of the IACUC, there are three critical issues that need to be addressed:

1. Have alternatives been considered? Can the educational objectives of students be met with computer simulations of cells, tissues, organs, and whole animals, including humans, videotapes, interactive videos, and nonanimal inanimate objects? If the use of animals is necessary, then the use of these methods beforehand may maximize the students' learning experience later when they start working with animals. Where feasible, assigning more than one student to an animal will reduce animal usage. Wherever possible, the IACUC should discourage killing vertebrate animals for educational purposes.

2. The IACUC must ensure that the animals used for instructional purposes in classrooms or laboratories receive the same humane care and treatment as those used for research purposes, and that proper animal procedures are followed.[4, 24] Students should receive appropriate supervision, instructions, and training for the laboratory exercises assigned. For invasive procedures, this can include special aspects of anesthesia and surgery, as well as the signs of pain exhibited by that species of animal and the methods for alleviating such pain. There should be some means of obtaining student evaluations after the laboratory exercises.

3. There should be clearly written and well-publicized policies pertaining to the use of animals in teaching programs.[7, 24] Some students refuse to take part in academic exercises involving either live or dead animals. For those faculty who teach such laboratory exercises, it is essential to have an alternate activity for students who decline to participate for ethical reasons. Another strategy is simply to separate the laboratory experience as an elective course. Academic institutions, in conjunction with their IACUCs, should consider having written policies on student participation in exercises involving animals, including any available alternatives and the potential penalties, if any, for failure to participate.

4.12   ESTABLISHMENT OF SATELLITE FACILITIES

At academic centers where research programs and faculty are constantly changing, occasionally a situation arises in which a faculty member or department wants to set up a new animal holding area separate from the existing facilities. The motivation for establishing a new satellite facility may simply be for investigator convenience, but there may be more compelling reasons. Because the IACUC has the responsibility for inspecting animal holding areas for compliance with various laws and regulations, it should play an advisory role during all phases of planning. The institution may establish the need for a new facility, but the IACUC and AV should be consulted on its construction. Failure to do so might result in the facility falling short of mandated regulations and approved standards.

4.13   ANIMAL RESEARCH AT OTHER INSTITUTIONS

Because animal research projects can be extremely complex, a single researcher may depend upon other researchers or personnel for the completion of part, or even all, of the animal work. If this collaborative effort is available at the same institution, then the regulatory issues that need to be addressed by the IACUC are relatively straightforward. However, many times the animal procedures need to be conducted at another academic institution or private company. This raises the issue of shared responsibility for the animal research.[20] It is important that the IACUC identify these off-campus components of an animal project and obtain enough information to ensure the other facility has an adequate animal care and use program in place to conduct the animal work. This is easily accomplished by incorporating a question into the protocol form. As part of the protocol review process, the IACUC should request documentation that the other facility's IACUC has reviewed and approved its component of the animal project. The IACUC should also obtain a copy of the approved proposal, the facility's USDA registration number, the facility's OPRR assurance number, and AAALAC status. This issue, while clearly relevant for collaborative or subgranting academic institutions, also applies to animal dealers that perform surgery on animals as a necessary part of a proposed animal activity and companies that produce customized antibodies.[3, 25]

4.14 ASSURANCE OF PROTOCOL ADHERENCE

Principal investigators must comply with a wide array of local, state, and federal laws, regulations by funding agencies, institutional policies, and written contracts, in addition to their own animal-use protocols. Infractions of any of these may be accidental or intentional, and may range from the trivial oversight to gross neglect. When faced with such violations, there are key watershed decisions. The first is whether the problem needs to be brought to the IACUC's attention. Many, if not most, of the problems are of such a nature that they can be handled at the local level by the veterinary staff without giving notice to the IACUC. For those situations which fall into the gray zone, it may be prudent for the AV to at least alert the IACUC chair of the problem and ask for further guidance. However, if the problem centers around gross protocol noncompliance or mistreatment of animals, the IACUC must become involved. As required by the AWA, the IACUC should have procedures in place for handling allegations of noncompliance or mistreatment. These procedures should address the following questions.[10, 26]

4.14.1 WHAT CONSTITUTES PROTOCOL NONCOMPLIANCE?

The IACUC should have definitions or guidelines of mistreatment or noncompliance. Mistreatment is defined as wrongful or abusive physical or psychological treatment of an animal. Noncompliance implies someone is not following an approved procedure or policy. Examples include failure to follow terms and conditions of an approved protocol, housing animals in unapproved facilities, or beginning research projects without IACUC approval. Perhaps the best litmus test is, "Were animals adversely impacted and was this a significant departure from the approved protocol?" (See Chapter 12, Ethics and Quandaries.)

4.14.2 WHO CAN FILE A COMPLAINT WITH THE IACUC?

There should be no restrictions as to who can make an allegation. Complaints may come from the public, research staff, or other facility personnel. The AWA regulations mandate that personnel should be taught how to report a possible violation; there should be no implication that reporting an incident will be detrimental to the individual's standing within the organization. Ideally, all complaints brought to the IACUC are fully documented in writing and signed, but the IACUC should be prepared to investigate all complaints regardless of how they are reported. The committee may vote not to act on spurious, undocumented allegations, but must follow up on documented allegations with substance.

4.14.3   Who Should Investigate Allegations?

If the IACUC chair or the full committee has determined that there is sufficient cause to proceed with an investigation, then an investigative group should be formed. This may consist of one person, an IACUC subcommittee, or the full IACUC. There can also be non-IACUC members or consultants to provide necessary expertise or to represent interested parties.

4.14.4   How Should the Investigation Be Conducted?

The policies and procedures for conducting an investigation must respect due process and confidentiality for everyone involved to garner broad support for subsequent findings and actions that the IACUC may implement. Before beginning an investigation, the group should inform all persons involved about its purpose, confidentiality issues, and the intended procedures. The alleged violators must be informed and given every opportunity to present their positions. The investigative group should not presume mistreatment or noncompliance.

4.14.5   What Should Be Done with the Investigative Findings?

The result of the investigation is usually presented as a written report to the full IACUC with recommendations for action. Following review and discussion, the recommendations or modifications thereof, are then voted upon. Regardless of the outcome, the IO should be informed of the final IACUC findings and the actions if any, that will be taken.

The second major watershed decision deals with the course of action that the IACUC takes should it conclude that noncompliance has occurred. Short of stopping the research, and assuming the problem has been corrected, a range of in-house responses is possible, including written warnings, reprimands, required additional training, or suspension of certain privileges for a set time. However, the IACUC has legal authority to stop a research project, either temporarily or permanently, if there is serious or continuing noncompliance. This must be done at a convened meeting of a quorum with a suspension vote of a majority of the quorum present.[1, 2] If this happens, then a cascade of events must follow that includes the prompt notification of the OPRR, if the project is supported by the PHS, and the USDA, if it involves a regulated species.[20] Obviously, such external reporting has serious implications for everyone. A faculty member is likely to be devastated, yet this action may be necessary.

Further, in an academic institution, the IO can initiate additional disciplinary action involving academic oversight authorities (e.g., faculty ethics or senate committees). All of this certainly will impact on the investigator's research progress and professional career. In the case of a junior faculty member, such an incident may seriously jeopardize pursuit of tenure.[27] Finally, because such a situation may draw the attention of the media, the institution might consider formulating a policy about making public statements concerning such an investigation.

As difficult as these are, it is important to remember that, for whatever reason, if the in-house oversight process does not work, outside agencies with legal standing can become involved. This may result in stopping research, withholding of research funds at the level of the investigator or the whole institution, revocation of the institution's Letter of Assurance (LOA) and monetary fines.

Fortunately, incidents of mistreatment or noncompliance are not common. When they do occur, those responsible must approach the incident with the utmost concern for animal and human welfare.[10, 26] Addressing complaints is difficult, and an IACUC with a clear set of guidelines can act thoughtfully and systematically. If emotions become heightened, the IACUC may forget due process, make legal errors, and compromise confidential information. The fact that reputations and careers are on the line makes a responsible investigation essential. The IACUC has powerful authority given to it by federal law and, therefore, must carefully exercise its judgment when there is an accusation of mistreatment or noncompliance.

4.15   SUNSHINE LAWS

Sunshine laws include both federal and state laws that require that the public have access to certain records and that certain meetings be open to the public.[7, 28, 29] The Freedom of Information Act (FOIA, 5 USC 552) compels federal agencies to release official documents—except in a few specific cases pertaining to national security, federal investigations, and personnel information. The provisions of this Act apply to both AWA and PHS policy; thus, nearly all material pertaining to animal care and use programs that are held by these agencies are obtainable through FOIA requests, including the USDA inspection reports and the institution's LOA. In fact, certain summary information pertaining to USDA inspection reports are available now through the Internet. It is incumbent upon the institution to ensure the accuracy of these reports. The only exceptions are cases of ongoing investigations into alleged violations of the AWA or PHS policy in which case all relevant documents are protected until the investigation is completed. At that time, the entire case file may be subject to release. Because of the FOIA, and in order to protect the institution, its programs, and its employees, it is prudent for institutions to ensure that information beyond that required is not provided to any federal agency. In addition, care should be taken to make sure that where information is available in federal reports any rebuttal material or information is made an integral part of the files.

Regarding state laws, all 50 states have open meeting laws, and some of these also mandate public access to certain records.[28] Obviously, these laws are particularly pertinent to academic institutions that receive state funding. At issue has been whether or not the state sunshine laws pertain to IACUC meetings and records. The right of the public to attend IACUC meetings under the open meeting laws has been highly controversial. Nationwide, the denial of requests to attend IACUC meetings has often led to legal suits. Decisions have gone both ways.[10] Because state laws vary on this issue, each institution should seek its own legal counsel.

4.16   COMPENSATION FOR SERVICE

An issue that gets very little attention within the academic community is the compensation for faculty who serve on an IACUC. Unlike most other committees established within a college or university, the IACUC is a legally mandated committee that demands a significant amount of time from its members. In an academic institution, because at least a few members are likely to be research faculty, it is very important that their administrative service be recognized by their supervisors. Because these individuals are often on a tenure track, they should not be penalized for taking time from their research and teaching to serve on the IACUC. They should be rewarded.

Another form of compensation that might be considered is partial salary support. As a necessary administrative overhead expense, it would be commendable to cover a portion of a faculty member's salary while serving on the IACUC. The IO should support this policy.

4.17   EXTERNAL REVIEW

While IACUCs must conduct reviews of their policies and procedures at least every six months, they themselves are also subject to a variety of external reviews. These can be of two types. Most are compliance-oriented reviews such as those conducted by the USDA and AAALAC. They focus on regulatory compliance and highlight those items that are noncompliant. However, some institutions, particularly academic ones, periodically invite outside consultants to evaluate aspects of the animal care program, including the IACUC, not so much from a compliance perspective but more from an efficiency or scientific perspective. For example, in the context of the IACUC, the protocol review procedures might be examined to see if a more efficient though still compliant method could be used. These outside reviews usually result in a final report that may suggest new or innovative operative procedures. Such periodic consultations provide a different assessment beyond the issue of compliance, and may provide both short-term and long-term goals for improving the program's quality.

4.18   CONCLUSIONS

In principle, the role of the IACUC in an academic institution is no different from that in other types of research organizations. However, there are operational challenges that academic IACUCs must face to ensure that the institution is compliant with all relevant laws and regulations while also striving to avoid unnecessary delays in appropriate animal research and teaching projects. Top level leadership's commitment to a high quality animal care and use program will determine how successful the institution will be in achieving this balance.

REFERENCES

1. Animal Welfare Act, Pub. L. 99-198, 9 CFR (Parts 1, 2, and 3), 1985.
2. Public Health Service, Public Health Service Policy on Humane Care and Use of Laboratory Animals, U.S. Department of Health and Human Services, Washington, D.C., reprinted 1996.
3. Potkay, S., Garnett, N. L., Miller, J. G., Pond, C. L., and Doyle, D. J., Frequently asked questions about the Public Health Service policy on humane care and use of laboratory animals, *Contemp. Top.*, 36, 47, 1997.
4. Recommendations for Governance and Management of Institutional Animal Resources, Association of American Medical Colleges and Association of American Universities, 1985.
5. USDA Policy Number 15—IACUC Membership, April 14, 1997.
6. Raub, W. F., Cutting red tape on research, *Iss. Sci. Tech.*, Winter, 75, 1989.
7. *Institutional Administrator's Manual for Laboratory Animal Care and Use,* Public Health Service, NIH publication 88-2959.
8. *Guide for the Care and Use of Laboratory Animals,* National Research Council, National Academy Press, Washington, D.C., 1996.
9. Stricklin, W. R. and Mench, J. A., Oversight of the use of agricultural animals in university teaching and research, *ILAR News,* Winter, 9, 1994.
10. *Institutional Animal Care and Use Committee Guidebook,* Public Health Service, NIH publication 92-3415.
11. Swanson, J. C., Oversight of farm animals in research, *Lab. Animal,* 27, 28, 1998.
12. *Guide for the Care and Use of Agricultural Animals in Agricultural Research and Teaching,* Federation of American Societies of Food Animal Science, Savoy, IL, 1988.
13. Martin, T., Ethical wildlife research: the need for a team approach, *Contemp. Top.,* 36, 43 (abstr), 1997.
14. American Society of Ichthyologists and Herpetologists, Guidelines for use of fishes in field research, *Fisheries,* 13, 16, 1988.
15. American Society of Ichthyologists and Herpetologists, Guidelines for use of live amphibians and reptiles in field research, asih@mail.utexas.edu, accessed August 13, 1997.
16. American Ornithologists' Union, Guidelines for the use of wild birds in research, *Auk,* 105 (1, suppl), 1A, 1988.
17. Acceptable field methods in mammalogy: preliminary guidelines approved by the American Society of Mammologists, *J. Mammo.* 68, (4, suppl) 1, 1987.
18. farol@nersp.nerdc.ufl.edu, accessed February 12, 1998.
19. Garnett, N. L. and DeHaven, W. R., OPRR and USDA/Animal Care response on applicability of the animal welfare regulations and the PHS policy to dead animals and shared tissues, *Lab. Animal,* 26, 21, 1997.
20. Potkay, S., Garnett, N. L. Miller, J. G. et al., Frequently asked questions about the public health service policy on humane care and use of laboratory animals, *Lab. Animal,* 26, 24, 1995.
21. Prentice, E. D., Crouse, D. A., and Mann, M. D., Scientific merit review: the role of the IACUC, *ILAR News,* 34, 15, 1992.
22. jtannbm@sprynet.com, accessed February 27, 1997.
23. *Occupational Health and Safety in the Care and Use of Research Animals,* National Research Council, National Academy Press, Washington, D.C., 1997.
24. Hamm, T. E. Jr. and Blum, J. R., The humane use of animals in teaching, *Contemp. Top.,* 31, 20, 1992.

25. USDA Policy Number 16—Dealers Selling Surgically-Altered Animals to Researchers, April 14, 1997.
26. Silverman, J., IACUC handling of mistreatment or noncompliance, *Lab. Animal,* 23, 30, 1994.
27. pctillman@ucdavis.edu, accessed August 22, 1996.
28. Orlans F. B., *In the Name of Science—Issues in Responsible Animal Experimentation,* Oxford University Press, New York, 1993.
29. *The Biomedical Investigator's Handbook for Researchers Using Animal Models,* Foundation for Biomedical Research, Washington, D.C., 1987.

5 Forms and Notices (Annotated)

M. Lawrence Podolsky, M.D.

CONTENTS

5.1 THE APPLICATION OR PROTOCOL FORM

Federal regulations state that all individuals and institutions covered by the Animal Welfare Act must "make, keep, and maintain systems of records or forms which fully and correctly disclose" all pertinent information about the use and disposition of animals under their jurisdiction.* Both the USDA and PHS mandate that all activities involving animals must be described in a protocol, which has to be reviewed and approved by an IACUC before any work with animals begins. A protocol, therefore, not only spells out the details of a proposed activity, but, in essence, serves as a contract between the animal user and the IACUC: it must be clear, specific, and understood by both sides.

There are no official templates for protocols. This is not an oversight, but rather a means of allowing the scientific community to enjoy some flexibility in meeting performance standards. It also permits adaptations to deal with a wide variety of animals. As a consequence, a diverse assortment of forms were invented—some as short as a half page memo, others as long as a booklet. In the latter category, as regulations and policies changed, additional sections were added onto existing protocol forms.

---

*AWA regulations do not mention *protocols*, hence *application* is sometimes used in the title.

0-8493-2580-3/99/$0.00+$.50
© 1999 by CRC Press LLC

Protocol documents from universities, pharmaceutical companies, and research laboratories were collected by this author, then integrated into the following generic form. Because these documents varied to reflect particular types of research or teaching, and covered all forms of life from invertebrates up to large zoo animals and non-human primates, the following conventions were used to show what should be printed on the form and what explanations or guidance would be useful to those filling out the form. The main headings are **numbered and appear in bold type.** Items that should be printed alongside the main headings are <u>underlined</u> (but on your institutional form these should not be underlined). Matter that should be addressed under this heading appear in regular type. *Comments and qualitative or annotating material appear in italics.*

The protocol is divided into six sections:

Section I: General information that identifies the institution, the personnel involved, and an overview of the project.
Section II: Number of animals that will be used and appropriateness of species.
Section III: Surgical and nonsurgical procedures.
Section IV: Alternative consideration and literature search.
Section V: Statement of assurances.
Section VI: IACUC actions.

5.2   SAMPLE PROTOCOL FORM

SECTION I

1. **NAME OF COMPANY/INSTITUTION/ORGANIZATION.** Only Name and Logo are needed here. *Because this document is for "internal use only," addresses, phone and fax numbers, and other logistical infomation may or may not be added.*

2. **AUTHORITY.** INSTITUTIONAL ANIMAL CARE AND USE COMMITTEE. Some forms carry this additional statement: <u>Federal animal welfare regulations require that the Institutional Animal Care and Use Committee (IACUC) must review and approve activities involving the use of vertebrate animals prior to their initiation. This includes animals used for experimental method development or for instructional purposes. In addition, approved protocols for ongoing activities must be reviewed by the IACUC at least annually.</u>

   Most seasoned investigators are trained to understand the duties and functions of IACUCs so there is no need for this statement. Where there is a rapid turnover in researchers or an influx of people from other sites and other countries, this serves as a steady reminder.

At universities and other institutions where grants provide funding for research, the following section is generally included. (See Chapter 4 for more on Academia.)

Protocols and Grants

Most, but not all, granting agencies allow one to apply for a grant before the protocol has been approved. If your protocol has been submitted, but is not yet approved, indicate to the granting agency that the protocol is "pending." NIH and NSF normally allow 60 days for approval. If the IACUC fails to approve your protocol within 60 days of the deadline date for the grant application, the agency may discard your grant application.

Some funding agencies (such as the American Heart Association) require that the protocol be approved before the grant is submitted. Investigators are responsible for knowing the requirements of their particular agency.

3. **TITLE OF THE DOCUMENT.** *This should read:* PROTOCOL FOR THE HUMANE CARE AND USE OF LIVE VERTEBRATE ANIMALS or IACUC ANIMAL USE REQUEST FORM. *The date of introduction or date of the most recent revision of this form should appear as a footer in the lowest left-hand corner.*

4. **PROTOCOL NUMBER** *After IACUC approval is granted.*

    DATE SUBMITTED *Not essential but helpful in resolving complaints about long delays.*

    DATE APPROVED *This may be placed on cover page for easy record keeping or may be placed at the end of the document next to the signatures of the chair or reviewers.*

5. **PROTOCOL TITLE.** Briefly state procedures to be carried out and the animal species to be used.
    Examples:
    HEALTH MONITORING OF GUINEA PIGS (for screenings of vendor animals and breeding colonies).
    EVALUATION OF DRUG(S) FOR OSTEOPOROSIS IN SQUIRREL MONKEYS (for drug screening and analytical studies).
    TISSUE HARVEST IN RATS (for specific organs or tissues).
    EXPERIMENTAL COMPOUNDS: TOXICITY STUDIES IN DOGS (a prerequisite for drug approval).
    MONOCLONAL ANTIBODY PRODUCTION IN RABBITS (for making and collecting specific antibodies).
    PRODUCTION OF TRANSGENIC AND GENE KNOCKOUT MICE (for genetic manipulations).

6. MULTIPLE USES. WILL ANIMALS USED UNDER THIS PROTO-
   COL BE USED UNDER OTHER PROTOCOLS? (CHECK) YES
   OR NO
   IF YES, STATE PROTOCOL TITLE AND NUMBER, DESCRIBE
     ASSOCIATION
   *(Example: Investigator A filled out a protocol to make animals hyper-
   tensive by means of renal surgery. Investigator B now wants to test
   research compounds for their antihypertensive effects on these same
   animals. A new protocol is needed because the first one only covered
   surgery. Investigator B would check off YES and describe the association.)*

7. **PRINCIPAL INVESTIGATOR.** NAME, ADDRESS, PHONE
   NUMBER *(Location and phone numbers facilitate communications
   between IACUC and applicant.)*

8. **DEPARTMENT AND BUSINESS UNIT or COURSE or PROJECT.**

9. **PERSONNEL INVOLVED** (other than veterinary services and people who normally provide animal care). Everyone working on this
   protocol must initial and date it to verify that they have read it and will
   comply with procedures described. Alternatively, a statement may be
   included that places full responsibility on the principal investigator for
   ensuring that everyone working on the project will comply with all procedures described in the protocol.

   Name   Phone Extension   Mail Stop   Initial and Date

10. **BRIEF SUMMARY.** Summarize proposed use of animals, including
    the purpose and nature of the use or experiment, time sequence of
    related procedures, and final disposition of animals. For resubmissions,
    state what has been accomplished under this protocol so far. Please
    define acronyms and abbreviations. *This section may appear redundant
    in view of the detailed information that follows, but it can be extremely
    helpful in understanding a series of complex procedures if the overall
    picture can be viewed ahead of time. Emphasis: this must be written in
    layperson's language. It should not be a "cut and paste" excerpt from
    a grant proposal.*

SECTION II

11A. **ANIMALS TO BE USED IN THIS PROTOCOL**
     SPECIES:
     SEX:
     AGE or WEIGHT RANGE:
     NUMBER OF ANIMALS TO BE USED ANNUALLY:

11B. EXPLAIN HOW THIS NUMBER WAS DETERMINED: *(It is helpful to have the input from a biostatistician here to justify the number of animals needed for statistically significant results. Avoid unnecessary duplications.*

11C. PROVIDE A RATIONALE FOR INVOLVING ANIMALS, AND FOR THE APPROPRIATENESS OF THE SPECIES.

12. **SOURCE.** Bred in-house or purchased from vendor.

13. **HUSBANDRY**
Standard Laboratory Animal Resource husbandry *(routine)*.
Specialized or nonlaboratory animal resource husbandry (described below) (often necessary for surgically altered animals, for special light cycles, special diets, deviations from psychological enrichments, and other departures from standard veterinary practice).

14. **PLAN FOR POSITIVE HUMAN INTERACTION.** If dogs or primates are used in experiments that last more than one day, describe your plan to provide positive human interaction above the standard.

SECTION III

15. **EXPERIMENTAL ADMINISTRATIONS/NONSURGICAL PROCEDURES.** List precisely the agent(s), adjuvants, vehicle, route of administration, volume (expressed in appropriate units), frequency of dosing (expressed as number of times a day), and duration of dosing. See Appendix I, Volume Guidelines for Compound Administration.

Agent	Dose (mg/kg)	Route	Frequency	Duration

16A. **SURGERY.** NO (Proceed to **18**).
YES. Check appropriate box:
❑ Nonsurvival surgery: animals euthanized without regaining consciousness.
❑ Minor survival surgery: no penetration of a major body cavity.
❑ Major survival surgery: penetration of a major body cavity, or surgical alteration that results in permanent physical impairment.
DESCRIBE SURGERY IN DETAIL. You may use a separate attachment.

16B. LOCATION. Where will surgery be performed? Aseptic surgery area? Other (specify location).

16C. MONITORING AND SUPPORTIVE CARE. Preoperative and intraoperative.

17A. ANESTHESIA/ANALGESIA/TRANQUILIZERS. Describe in the boxes below the agents that may be used in:
   a) Surgical procedures.
   b) Other procedures. (This requires consultation with a veterinarian prior to submission.)

Agent	Dose (mg/kg)	Route	Frequency

17B. CRITERIA TO ASSESS LEVEL OF ANESTHESIA. Check all that apply.
   ❑ Respiration rate
   ❑ Heart rate
   ❑ ECG
   ❑ Toe pinch
   ❑ Tail pinch
   ❑ Corneal reflex
   ❑ Color of mucous membranes
   ❑ Muscular relaxation
   ❑ Other (pulse oximeter, respirometer)

17C. ANESTHESIA RECOVERY MONITORING. Survival procedures only. Will analgesia be provided?

17D. POSTSURGICAL RECOVERY MONITORING. Beyond anesthetic recovery.

18. BLOOD COLLECTIONS. Will blood be collected from animals? If NO, proceed to next section. If YES, then state METHOD, FREQUENCY, and VOLUME OF EACH WITHDRAWAL. Also state the estimated percentage of total volume withdrawn per day or week. See Appendix H, Guidelines for Blood Sample Withdrawal.

19. RESTRAINTS. Will unanesthetized animals be restrained (exclude momentary procedures such as for blood draws, injections, dosing, etc.? If NO, proceed to next section. If YES, then state purpose/method/duration/and frequency. Also describe how animals will be observed during periods of restraint, and what training/acclimatization procedures are to be carried out beforehand.

20. **FOOD AND WATER.** <u>Will food be withheld for more than 24 h or water for more than 8 h? If YES, state purpose/duration/and monitoring procedure.</u> *This can be tricky. Many animals are nocturnal; does the clock start ticking at the start of a working day or when the anima begins its activities?*

21. **REMOVAL FROM NORMAL ANIMAL FACILITIES.** <u>Will animals be kept in areas outside of the animal facilities for more than a working day?</u>
If YES describe location, length of time, and reason.
There must be strong reasons for taking animals away from strictly controlled animal facilities and placing them in highly variable laboratory environments.

22. **HAZARDOUS AGENTS.** <u>Will animals be subjected to any hazardous agents such as pathogenic organisms, chemical carcinogens, recombinant DNA/RNA, or radioactivity? Will animals be a source of contamination to personnel or other animals? If YES, describe agent(s), risks, how they will be used, containment procedures, and precautions for proper disposal of animals and waste. Also, document authorization or clearance from health and safety departments, if applicable.</u>

23. **EUTHANASIA.** <u>State the agent, dose (mg/kg), and route of administration of substances that will be used for euthanasia of test animals and moribund animals.</u>
<u>If this does not comply with the recommendations of the AVMA Panel on Euthanasia, provide justification.</u> See Appendix J, Euthanasia Guidelines.

24. **CRITERIA USED TO ASSESS PAIN/DISTRESS/DISCOMFORT.**
<u>Check all that apply:</u>
❑ Loss of appetite.
❑ Loss of weight.
❑ Restlessness.
❑ Abnormal resting postures in which the animal appears to be sleeping or is hunched up.
❑ Licking, biting, scratching, or shaking a particular area.
❑ Failure to show normal patterns of inquisitiveness.
❑ Failure to groom, causing an unkempt appearance.
❑ Guarding (protecting the painful area).
❑ Loss of mobility.
❑ Red stain around the eyes of rats.
❑ Unresponsiveness.
❑ Self-mutilation.
❑ Labored breathing.
❑ Other.

It is not necessary to list every sign of pain or distress, however, such a list serves as a constant reminder and educational tool.

25. **LIMITING PAIN AND DISCOMFORT TO ANIMALS.** Describe procedures designed to assure that discomfort and pain will be limited to that which is unavoidable for the conduct of scientifically valid research.

26. **ALTERNATIVES.** Consideration of alternatives to each procedure that may cause pain or distress must state sources consulted, such as BIOLOGICAL ABSTRACTS, INDEX MEDICUS, MEDLINE, AGRICOLA, EMBASE, BIOSIS, LIFE SCIENCES, ZOOLOGICAL RECORD, ASFA, PSYCHINFO, TOXLINE, CAB, ARIS, PASCAL, THE CURRENT RESEARCH INFORMATION SERVICE (CRIS), and the Animal Welfare Information Center (AWIC). The minimal written narrative should include the databases searched or other sources consulted, the date of the search and the years covered by the search, and the key words and/or search strategy used by the Principal Investigator when considering alternatives or descriptions of other methods and sources used to determine that no alternatives were available to the painful or distressful procedure. The narrative should be such that the IACUC can readily assess whether the search topics were appropriate and whether the search was sufficiently thorough. Reduction, replacement, and refinement (the three Rs) must be addressed, not just animal replacement.
See Appendix C, Directory for Alternatives, and Appendix D, Major Databases.

27. **PRINCIPAL INVESTIGATOR STATEMENT OF ASSURANCE:** Check the appropriate answer, YES or NO. (Note: A negative answer to any statement requires a detailed, written explanation.)

YES	NO	
❑	❑	No animal will be used in more than one major operative procedure from which it is allowed to recover, unless scientifically justified or required as a veterinary procedure.
❑	❑	Paralytics will not be used without appropriate anesthesia.
❑	❑	Medical care for animals will not be withheld and will be available and provided or supervised as necessary by a veterinarian.
❑	❑	The animals' living conditions, including housing, feeding, psychological enrichment programs, exercise, and nonmedical care, will be appropriate for the species, will contribute to their health and comfort, and will not deviate from USDA Standards.
❑	❑	Animals that would otherwise experience severe or chronic pain/distress that cannot be relieved will be euthanized at the end of the procedure, or if appropr during the procedure.
❑	❑	Personnel conducting animal procedures will be appropriately qualified and trained in those procedures, and

the training and qualifications of such personnel will

_____   _____

_____   _____

_____   _____

_____

_____

_____

_____   _____

_____   _____

EXPERIMENTAL COMPOUNDS: TOXICITY STUDIES IN DOGS (a
prerequisite for drug approval).
MONOCLONAL ANTIBODY PRODUCTION IN RABBITS (for making
and collecting specific antibodies).
PRODUCTION OF TRANSGENIC AND GENE KNOCKOUT MICE (for
genetic manipulations).
**Questions 11, 25, and 26 should reflect your efforts to refine the proce-
dures, to reduce the number of animals used, and to replace them when
possible.** REFINEMENT of procedures requires the utilization of all modalities
that will decrease pain and/or distress in animals—from psychological enrichment to appropriate use of analgesics. (IACUC performs inspections of ongoing protocols which often result in refinements.) REDUCTION means using
just enough animals to give statistically significant results. REPLACEMENT
requires the consideration of computer modeling, cell cultures, nonanimal
insentient materials, nonmammalian or invertebrate species instead of mammalian animals

- **Question 11B: Estimate Number of Animals/Explain How This
  Number Was Determined:** Investigators are encouraged to consult with
  statisticians and information specialists in making this determination.
  Avoid all unnecessary duplications.
- **Question 11C: Provide a Rationale for Involving Animals and for the
  Appropriateness of the Species.** See next section for guidance.
- **Question 26: Provide a Written Narrative of Alternatives.** When look-
  ing for alternatives to procedures that may cause pain or distress or the
  replacement of mammalian animals, investigators must state sources con-
  sulted, such as BIOLOGICAL ABSTRACTS, INDEX MEDICUS, MED-
  LINE, AGRICOLA, EMBASE, BIOSIS, LIFE SCIENCES,
  ZOOLOGICAL RECORD, ASFA, PSYCHINFO, TOXLINE, CAB, ARIS
  PASCAL, THE CURRENT RESEARCH INFORMATION SERVICE
  (CRIS), and the Animal Welfare Information Center (AWIC). Additionally
  investigators may restate information gathered from networking and col-
  laboration with colleagues, and from local, regional, and national scien-
  tific/professional meetings where new techniques, equipment, and/or
  models were presented. The minimal written narrative should include the
  databases searched or other sources consulted, the date of the search, the
  years covered by the search, and the key words and/or search strategy. The
  narrative should be such that the IACUC can readily assess whether the
  search topics were appropriate and whether the search was sufficiently
  thorough.

5.3   PROTOCOL AMENDMENT

If every detail of every experiment was known beforehand, there would be no need
for the experiment. But, because there are many unknowns, it is often necessary to

modify a protocol as work progresses. The best way to handle this is through the **Protocol Amendment.** This should be simple and straightforward.

1. **NAME OF ORGANIZATION.**
2. **TITLE OF DOCUMENT.** Institutional Animal Care and Use Committee PROTOCOL AMENDMENT.
3. **DATE SUBMITTED.**
4. **PROTOCOL NUMBER.**
5. **PROTOCOL TITLE.**
6. **USDA CLASSIFICATION.**
7. **PRINCIPAL INVESTIGATOR..**
8. **CHANGES TO BE MADE.** Applicant should note which section(s) of the original approved protocol are to be changed, restate the original wording, then state the new wording to reflect the changes needed.
9. **REASONS FOR CHANGES.**
10. **PERSONNEL CHANGES.** Delete the names of personnel no longer associated with this protocol and add names that were not on the original protocol.

Whether new and old personnel sign this amendment is discretionary. Regulatory and administrative policies and procedures do not address requirement. Some IACUCs feel that everyone affected by the protocol should know about the modifications and should show their awareness about them by signing the amendment.

SIGNATURE(S) OF PRINCIPAL INVESTIGATOR(S)   **DATE**

APPROVED BY   **DATE**

VETERINARIAN Applies to Category D and E protocols.   **DATE**

A footer in the lower left-hand corner
states the date of most recent revision of this form.

Many IACUCs have voted to permit the chair to approve amendments to protocols classified as C, but insist that the full IACUC review and approve amendments to E protocols. Amendments to D protocols may fall either way.

Sometimes it is necessary to amend an amendment. How should this be handled? As a rule, if the second amendment is minor (dealing with only one part of a section or with a minor technical adjustment), it may be handled just like the initial amendment. However, if the amended amendment is long, complicated, or otherwise changes procedures, dosages, surgery, restraints, or other controversial areas, it is usually better to submit a new protocol.

If the amendment changes the USDA pain category to a higher level, say from a C to a D or E, the IACUC may ask for a new protocol instead of an amendment.

The next three forms are issued and enforced by the IACUC chair and are discussed in other chapters.

5.4   ANNUAL IACUC PROTOCOL RENEWAL FORM

To: Name of Principal Investigator   Date:

From: IACUC Chair

Protocol Title:

Protocol Number:

UDSA Category:

The IACUC protocol specified above was approved on (Date) and now requires annual renewal. To maintain approval status, return this form, completed, and signed at least two weeks before the anniversary date. Check the appropriate box below.

❑   Delete protocol. It is no longer being used.

   or

❑   Renew this protocol. It will be used with **no** revisions.

If the protocol needs revisions, then a proper Protocol Amendment Form must be executed before the annual review. Some institutions require an annual progress update and an updated search for alternatives.

Delete the following individuals from the personnel approved to carry out this protocol:

Add the following individuals to the list of personnel qualified to carry out this protocol. Each individual must sign or initial by their name to verify that they have read this protocol and will comply with procedures as described.

_____   _____

Signature of Principal Investigator   Date

A footer in the lower left-hand corner
states the date of most recent revision of this form.

5.5 PROTOCOL EXPIRATION NOTICE

To: <u>Name of Principal Investigator</u> Date: _____
From: <u>IACUC Chair</u>

Protocol Title:

Protocol Number: Approval Date (mo/yr): _____
USDA Category:
This IACUC protocol will expire on _____.

To continue the activities covered by this protocol, a completely rewritten protocol must be submitted at least four weeks before the expiration date. An IACUC review is also required. Kindly sign this notice and return it with the protocol. A new protocol number will be issued at the time of approval.

❑ Check this box to delete this protocol if it is no longer used.

_____ _____

Signature of Principal Investigator Date

A footer in the lower left-hand corner
states the date of most recent revision of this form.

5.6 ANIMAL LIMITS NOTICE

To: <u>Name of principal investigator</u> Date: _____

From: <u>IACUC Chair</u>

This memorandum informs you that you have reached 80 percent of your annual estimated animal limit for the protocol listed below. If you need to increase this number, please send an IACUC amendment to me requesting a revised annual limit and a justification for the revision.

Protocol Title:

Protocol Number:

Species: **Limit:** **Number of animals purchase to date:**

Please contact me at (phone number or extension) for questions or comments.

A footer in the lower left-hand corner
states the date of most recent revision of this form.

5.7   IACUC SEMIANNUAL ANIMAL CARE AND USE PROGRAM REVIEW

Date of Review: _____

	Satisfactory	Unsatisfactory
A. INSTITUTIONAL POLICIES		
1. Monitoring the care and use of animals	_____	_____
2. Veterinary care	_____	_____
3. Personnel qualifications	_____	_____
4. Personnel hygiene	_____	_____
5. Occupational health program	_____	_____
6. Experimentation involving hazardous agents	_____	_____
7. Special considerations	_____	_____
B. LABORATORY ANIMAL HUSBANDRY		
1. Housing	_____	_____
2. Food	_____	_____
3. Bedding	_____	_____
4. Sanitation	_____	_____
5. Animal identification records	_____	_____
6. Experimentation involving hazardous agents	_____	_____
7. Provisions for emergency, weekend, and holiday care	_____	_____
C. VETERINARY CARE		
1. Preventive medicine	_____	_____
2. Surveillance, diagnosis, treatment, and control of animal diseases	_____	_____
3. Anesthesia and analgesia	_____	_____
4. Survival surgery and postsurgical care	_____	_____
5. Euthanasia	_____	_____
D. PHYSICAL PLANT		
1. Overview of general arrangement and condition of facility	_____	_____
2. Functional space	_____	_____
3. Support areas	_____	_____
4. General features of animal rooms	_____	_____
5. Other features	_____	_____
E. SPECIAL CONSIDERATIONS		
1. Genetics and nomenclature	_____	_____
2. Facilities and procedures for animal research involving hazardous agents	_____	_____

OVERALL PROGRAM REVIEW:

Comments:

_____
_____
_____

Follow-up required: /

_____
_____
_____

Dissenting opinions:

_____
_____
_____

IACUC MEMBERS (signatures)

_____ _____ _____

A footer in the lower left-hand corner
states the date of most recent revision of this form.

5.8 ANIMAL FACILITY SEMIANNUAL INSPECTION REPORT FORM

This is NOT an all-inclusive form. It is a sample of one way to report findings of a semiannual inspection. Every institution should design a form that covers its own particular facilities.

DATE: _____

FACILITY	OK	Needs Work	Major	Minor	Comments	Correction	Date
Cage wash—dirty							
Cage wash—clean							
Feed storage							
Shower room							
General storage							
Mouse room							
Hepa-filtered room							
Recovery/animal							
Surgeon prep room							
Surgery room							
Rabbit/rodent							
Equipment room							
Preclinical lab							
Outer corridor							
Animal corridor							

IACUC Member making this report:

Other IACUC Members present during this inspection:

A footer in the lower left-hand corner
states the date of most recent revision of this form.

5.9 PROTOCOL POINTERS

Protocol forms may be distributed as printed forms, photocopies, or presented on a university or corporate network, or on other electronic media (web page) for downloading, as necessary.

Protocols are reviewed annually and must be rewritten and resubmitted every three years.

Protocols may be reviewed by a subcommittee of the IACUC or the committee as a whole; however, every member of the committee may call for a full review of any protocol at any time.

Upon annual review, protocols are extended for one year, provided there are no changes—other than personnel. If (substantive) changes are required, then the Protocol Amendment Form should be completed and acted upon prior to renewal.

When a person leaves one institution for another to continue the same work covered by an IACUC approved protocol, is it necessary to fill out a new protocol? Each IACUC is only responsible for research performed at their own institution. Also, it is a good idea to request one so that members of the new IACUC have the opportunity to review all facets of animal usage. Also, because new personnel will be involved at the new institution, a new protocol is needed. Indeed, the responsibilities of occupational health and safety are often met, in part, by identifying personnel in the protocol.

Investigators are often required to submit protocols to department or section heads, funding agencies, legal departments, or other corporate/academic bodies before experiments can be funded or authorized. Hence, there may be several procols under review simultaneously, for the same study. **The protocol before the IACUC takes precedence over all others.**

6 Running an IACUC: One Chair's Perspective

Victor S. Lukas, D.V.M.

CONTENTS

6.1   INTRODUCTION

Running an IACUC is a challenging task that requires diplomacy, attention to detail, and a determination to provide high standards for animal care and use. An effective IACUC not only facilitates research while ensuring animal welfare, but it also evaluates scientific methods related to animal use. Additionally, it makes recommendations for improving science. IACUCs are intended to be self-regulating bodies, and when necessary, enforce government regulations and institutional policies. *How* IACUCs actually function can mean the difference between collegial cooperative and adversarial counterproductive interactions. As Dr. Ben Cohen, one of the founding fathers of modern laboratory animal science would tell his students, "Find ways to say **yes.**" This chapter will discuss efficient and effective methods of running IACUCs based on that precept.

6.2   WHO IS ON FIRST BASE?

The intent of the USDA Animal Welfare Act (AWA) is to have the *legal buck* stop at the institutional official's desk. According to the AWA's definition, the "institutional official means the individual at a research facility who is authorized to certify that the requirements of 9 CFR Parts 1, 2, and 3, will be met." This individual, typically the chief executive officer or president, must appoint the IACUC chair and members. Our IACUC retains all memos from the institutional official that relate to membership changes. This serves as documentation that we are in compliance with the law.

A key component in the success of IACUCs and the programs they oversee is strong support from the IO. This can be demonstrated by the IO taking timely action when needed and committing resources when problems arise. When the program is running smoothly, periodic visits to IACUC meetings, occasional participation in facility inspections, and attendance at IACUC sponsored seminars are means of demonstrating strong IACUC support. At our institution, we invite the IO to the end of the year IACUC banquet that is held to show appreciation for the work by committee members. This gesture, offered in a relaxed, social setting is well received by all and provides the opportunity for the IO to personally thank everyone on behalf of the institution.

Typically, there are one to three key figures at each institution who run the IACUC—the chair, the attending veterinarian, and the coordinator/administrative assistant. At some institutions, there may be three individuals or one or two individuals with multiple responsibilities. This number depends upon such factors as the size of the institution, the percent of effort for each person who works on the IACUC, individual performance, and established operating procedures. Many committees create unnecessary work for themselves (see Chapter 3, IACUC Records and Their Management) and consequently, need to devote greater resources to operate.

The IACUC chair is typically the person who has the greatest impact on how an IACUC operates. Some institutions have created positions such as an executive secretary or administrator. This person performs many behind-the-scenes tasks normally associated with the chair. This arrangement limits the chair primarily to running meetings and serving as a committee spokesperson. It also provides continuity when the IACUC has a rotating chair (i.e., a chair that serves for a specified period, such as 12 months), or when the IO appoints a senior researcher who has only a limited amount of time to devote to the committee. For the purpose of this chapter, when we refer to the chair's responsibilities, that also implies an executive secretary's responsibilities.

The Association for Assessment and Accreditation of Laboratory Animal Care International (AAALAC) discourages animal care program directors from serving as IACUC chairs, owing to the "fox watching the henhouse" theory. Veterinarians, however, although not an ideal candidate at some institutions, may make good IACUC chairs. They are well-versed in regulations and policies, have a broad scientific education, and have a general knowledge of the animal research performed at their institution. A conflict of interest could arise if, for example, the IACUC discovered deficiencies in the veterinary program. It is important to remember that the chair does not possess any more authority than any other IACUC member. The committee as a whole, reporting to the IO, has the authority. An issue for veterinarians working on IACUCs, in general, is that researchers may be reluctant to report animal health problems to the veterinary staff, especially when adversarial relationships exist between researchers and the committee. This conflict is most likely to arise when veterinarians act as "IACUC policeman." When enforcement is necessary, it is preferred to have someone other than the veterinarian involved. If the veterinarian is the chair, then he or she must exercise extreme diplomacy.

6.3   WHO DOES WHAT?

The specific federally mandated IACUC functions are outlined in the Applied Research Ethics National Association (ARENA)/Office for Protection from Research Risks (OPRR) *Institutional Animal Care and Use Guidebook.*

Below are lists of general responsibilities for the IACUC chair, coordinator, and attending veterinarian at our institution. Those that are not directly linked to mandated IACUC functions are labeled as optional. These lists are provided as an illustration of how responsibilities can be delegated to several key individuals and also to demonstrate the complexity of IACUC functions. Documenting specific duties is also useful when there is turnover of these individuals at an institution. It minimizes confusion and prevents certain tasks, especially those that are only repeated annually, from falling between the cracks.

The chair's responsibilities include:

- Ensures compliance with IACUC-related USDA and PHS regulations, and AAALAC guidelines.
- Recommends membership change to the IO.
- Maintains a current principal investigator list.
- Convenes/chairs meetings; designates acting chair if unable to attend meeting; cancels meeting when no protocols are submitted.
- Ensures that a quorum is present to conduct meetings.
- Ensures that semiannual program reviews are performed every six months and appropriately documented. Takes appropriate action based on findings; submits reports to IO.
- Ensures adequate documentation of IACUC activities, such as meeting agendas, meeting minutes, inspection reports, and membership changes.
- Reviews and documents approval of protocols, amendments, and protocol renewals/deletions/expirations.
- Acts as spokesperson on behalf of the IACUC, both internally and externally.
- Represents the IACUC to USDA and Food and Drug Administration (FDA) inspectors and AAALAC site visitors.
- Directs IACUC expenditures, including donations and institutional memberships.
- Coordinates the IACUC subcommittees.
- Investigates cases of noncompliance and complaints about the care or use of laboratory animals. Depending on the severity of noncompliance, the IACUC may take actions such as requiring additional training or suspending the principal investigator's (PI) protocol.

The following are optional responsibilities:

- Prepares the OPRR Assurance Statement and annual reports.
- Prepares the USDA Annual Report of Research Facilities; submits report to the USDA Animal Care Regional Director by December 1 of each calendar year.

The IACUC coordinator's responsibilities include:

- Assists investigators and IACUC representatives in obtaining IACUC forms such as protocol and amendment forms.
- Screens new protocols for completeness and appropriate signatures.
- Schedules meeting times and locations for the entire year; sends a schedule to committee members, ex officio members, and principal investigators.
- Drafts a meeting agenda prior to each meeting. After the chair approves, the coordinator sends agenda and attachments to the committee.
- Once the meeting begins, takes meeting minutes that include, but are not limited to, attendance, review of protocols and amendments, and other committee decisions.
- After each meeting, reviews minutes with the chair. Once the chair approves the draft minutes, the coordinator sends the minutes to the committee and requests a review in five working days. The minutes are considered approved if no comments are received. If the minutes are significantly revised, they are resent to the committee for further review.
- After approval of a protocol, assigns a protocol number, sends an approval memo and a copy of the protocol to the principal investigator, enters information into the database, saves an electronic copy, and files the original copy.
- Maintains files of IACUC documents; archives inactive protocol files; destroys outdated documents not less than three years after they are generated, or for protocols and amendments, three years after cessation of the activity.
- Initiates/tracks annual protocol renewal forms and protocol expiration forms.
- Maintains computerized database for tracking activity of protocols.
- Initiates notification when an investigator reaches 80 percent of the annual limit of the number of animals an investigator is allowed to procure under a protocol; notifies the chair and the investigator if an animal order is placed that would exceed the approved limit.
- Distributes the current list of approved protocols, approximately monthly, to animal facility supervisors, to confirm that the correct protocol numbers are entered on animal order forms before submitting to the animal purchasing coordinator.

The following are optional responsibilities.

- Creates/distributes a monthly report of IACUC activities.
- Maintains files from organizations such as the California Biomedical Association, Foundation for Biomedical Research, Scientist Center for Animal Welfare, National Association for Biomedical Research, and so on.

The attending veterinarian's IACUC-related responsibilities include:

- Provides adequate veterinary care.
- Chairs the Animal Studies Inspection Subcommittee (see IACUC Subcommittees below for details).
- Provides veterinary review of USDA Category D and E protocols.
- Consults with researchers on subjects such as surgery, sedatives, analgesics, anesthetics, and euthanasia methods; recommends options for ensuring humane use of the animals while meeting the scientific requirements of the study.
- Consults with animal husbandry personnel, Occupational Health Services, and Environmental Health and Safety on issues such as animal nutrition, exercise, psychological enrichment, facility sanitation, zoonotic agents, hazardous agents, and so on.

6.4   IACUC MEMBERSHIP

Opinions differ on the ideal composition of an IACUC because an institution may be subject to three similar but differing requirements.

USDA—if an institution uses USDA-covered species, all warm-blooded animals except birds, rats, and mice (refer to the AWA definition of *animal*), the IACUC must have at least three members: a chairman, a doctor of veterinary medicine, and a person not affiliated with the facility. If the IACUC has more than three members, not more than three can be from the same administrative unit.

Public Health Service (PHS)—If an institution conducts PHS supported activities, then the IACUC must comply with the National Institutes of Health, OPRR *PHS Policy on Humane Care and Use of Laboratory Animals* (PHS policy). The committee must have at least five members that include a veterinarian as mentioned previously, a nonaffiliated person as mentioned previously, a practicing scientist experienced in animal research, and a nonscientist. An individual may fulfill more than one of these categories, for example, a nonaffiliated, nonscientist.

AAALAC—If an institution is also AAALAC accredited, then it must comply with the Institute of Laboratory Animal Resources (ILAR) *Guide for the Care and Use of Laboratory Animals.* By complying with the USDA and PHS regulations, it should be in compliance with this Guide. At least three members are required: a doctor of veterinary medicine, a practicing scientist experienced in animal research, and a nonaffiliated public member. Unlike the other two regulations, the Guide specifies that the public member should not be a laboratory animal user.

There are some IACUCs with over 20 members. Our IACUC has 11 members. To convene a meeting, a quorum, or a majority of the members, in our case six, must be present. To approve protocols or suspend an activity, the majority of the quorum must agree. The PHS policy states that an IACUC member who has a conflicting interest must not contribute to the quorum. To use our IACUC as an example, when we review a member's protocol, then that member must abstain from voting and may not be counted as one of the six members needed to establish a quorum for the purpose of reviewing his or her protocol. In other words, we would need at least seven members total to be present.

Our 11 person IACUC consists of the chair, a clinical veterinarian (also the Animal Studies Inspection Subcommittee Chair), 5 practicing scientists who work with animals, 2 nonaffiliated public members (a retired pediatrician and a high school science teacher), a biostatistician who also serves as our nonscientist, and the manager of the animal facilities (also the Facilities Subcommittee Chair). We also have three ex officio, nonvoting members: the director of the laboratory animal resources program, the director of the quality assurance unit, and the supervisor of the animal health technician staff (also the Training Subcommittee Chair). Other types of IACUC members who may be useful include ethicists, clergy, occupational health physicians or nurse practitioners, environmental health specialists, building engineers, husbandry staff, research assistants, lawyers, pathologists, humane society representatives, librarians, and so on. There are advantages and disadvantages for each type of member.

The qualities that contribute most toward making ideal IACUC members may not be related to their professions. Committee work is sometimes jokingly considered punishment for sins of a past life because it can be tedious and boring. Of course, most people would prefer the work to be interesting, educational, and occasionally fun. The difference frequently depends on the personality types of the members. Qualities that we consider desirable in IACUC members are first, a desire to promote the welfare of research animals, and second, to advance science. There should also be a willingness to freely express opinions while listening to opinions of others. Above all, IACUC members should be able to critically and logically evaluate issues without bias, and to "think out of the box" in order to suggest novel approaches to problems. On the practical side, it is helpful to have members who are well-organized and capable of adhering to deadlines. IACUCs impose many deadlines on researchers, therefore IACUCs should, in turn, respect other people's time.

These are the rules we try to instill in our team—rules that we attempt to implement when confronted by a disruptive IACUC member, or one with "needs improvement" (to be polite) personality traits.

- Do not monopolize discussions; encourage others to express their opinions.
- Do not interrupt.
- Be polite; do not distract others by whispering during discussions.
- Be respectful of researchers, do not induce resentment because you feel you have some authority over them.

This seems like common-sense advice, but we have witnessed these behaviors in IACUC meetings. They are unprofessional and counterproductive.

A problem occasionally encountered when forming an IACUC is choosing a nonaffiliated member. The difficulty is compounded by scheduling IACUC meetings during business hours, thereby requiring nonaffiliated members to leave their place of employment for several hours. To prevent the appearance of an institution influencing or biasing the nonaffiliated member, the work is either voluntary or, at best, basic expenses are paid. This provision alone discourages many hourly employees from serving on IACUCs. Finding an interested nonaffiliated member typically depends on networking with friends or acquaintances at church or a synagogue, or by contacting local organizations like veterinary or human medical associations, non-profit organizations such as the American Cancer Society, or responsible animal welfare groups. Owing to the sensitivity of issues discussed, choosing the nonaffiliated member is critically important. When the new member joins, help him/her feel welcome and encourage him/her to participate. If he/she has little prior experience, provide an orientation session or send him/her to training meetings. If he/she does not understand the issues and is unfamiliar with scientific writing, he/she may feel intimidated or insecure and will not contribute. Help him/her to be a productive member.

The practicing scientists serving on our IACUC are referred to as IACUC representatives. Each of the approximately 55 principal investigators (PIs) is assigned to one of these representatives. The representatives and their assigned PIs are usually from the same department or business unit. The representatives preview protocols and amendments from their PIs before submission to the IACUC, and they may present or defend the protocol during deliberations. The preview by the representatives and the veterinarian for USDA Category D and E protocols is an important step in the protocol review process. Numerous issues are clarified or resolved before reaching the full committee, thereby minimizing or eliminating unnecessary delays for researchers and reducing time spent in committee. Frequently, researchers misinterpret questions on the protocol form or unintentionally omit information. The veterinarian may propose better methods of anesthesia, analgesia, or different surgical procedures. The discussion of alternatives to potentially painful or distressful procedures is probably the single most misunderstood section in the protocol review process. More information is provided below in the Protocol Review section of this chapter and in Chapter 11, The Literature Search for Alternatives. It is rare that a protocol survives the entire review process with no modifications and the preview is the first step.

6.5 PROTOCOL REVIEW

Protocol review consumes the greatest amount of IACUC time at most institutions. This applies to the preview, distribution, individual member review, discussion during the meeting, revisions and proofing, obtaining signatures, logging into the meeting minutes and database, and filing the hard copies. There are virtually as many procedures for conducting protocol review as there are IACUCs. Fortunately, unlike the varying requirements for membership, requirements in the AWA and PHS Policy are consistent. These requirements also apply to significant changes in ongoing IACUC-approved activities, generally referred to as amendments. Individual IACUCs may define what is significant. At our institution, we consider any activity that affects the use of animals as significant. A personnel change is an example of an activity that we would not consider significant.

The minimum requirements for protocol review are as follows:

- Prior to IACUC review, each IACUC member shall be provided with a list of protocols to be reviewed.
- The written protocol shall be available to any IACUC member upon request.

- Any member may obtain, upon request, full committee review, that is, at a convened meeting of a quorum.
- Approval at a full committee meeting is granted with the agreement of a majority of the quorum present.
- If full committee review is not requested, at least one member of the IACUC, designated by the chair, reviews the protocols and has the authority to approve, require modifications, or request full committee review. This process has been termed designated member review.
- A member who has a conflicting interest may not be part of a quorum.

A true designated member review may be used at very large institutions where it is impractical for each IACUC member to review every protocol, or possibly at small institutions where the IACUC meets routinely only every six months. Our IACUC, like most, sends a complete protocol to each member. We typically e-mail protocols to internal members, and fax copies or send by overnight delivery to our community members. Security may be a concern when sending documents electronically outside the institution's network; however, additional security measures are available.

Time is always a commodity in short supply at research institutions. Sending IACUC documents electronically saves the IACUC coordinator's time and speeds delivery. Deadlines are an issue for every IACUC. Researchers often want approval tomorrow and IACUCs need at least a week, to perhaps a month or more, to distribute the protocols and to provide sufficient time for members to review them. Our deadline for including a protocol on a meeting agenda is one week, assuming that it has been prereviewed by an IACUC representative. We may, with good justification, reduce the deadline by a few days, providing the requirements listed previously are satisfied. Allowing researchers to routinely ignore deadlines negatively impacts the morale and effectiveness of IACUC members who have regular jobs and require adequate time to adequately read each protocol and amendment.

An additional advantage of requesting an electronic copy of the protocol along with the signed original protocol is that our IACUC can save it in a database for future reference by other investigators. Upon request, our IACUC coordinator e-mails electronic copies to the requestor so they can "cut and paste" relevant sections into their protocols, thereby saving them considerable time. As a courtesy, we typically ask permission from the original author before sending it to the requestor. This practice may be less common in academic settings where researchers may be competing for funds. At some companies, all approved protocols are located on a common server that is directly accessible to all researchers.

Institutions have sought ways to expedite the review process, especially in cases of genuine need. There are no exceptions to the AWA or PHS Policy, nor are there any provisions for an expedited review process. At many institutions, there may be procedures for shortening the standard review process, that is, the time from when a researcher delivers a protocol to the IACUC to the time approval is granted. Theoretically, a researcher could submit a signed protocol and send an electronic copy to the IACUC office, which in turn could e-mail at least the title to all IACUC members, and the entire protocol to a designated reviewer and request review the same day. This assumes that the members had an opportunity to request full committee review, and the reviewer is available and willing to read it when it arrives, and no comments are made. This is an extreme example that is impractical to routinely implement. At our institution, we do not routinely include USDA Category C protocols on full committee meeting agendas because they typically necessitate minimal discussion. We send C protocols to every IACUC member with a request for comments in five working days, and consider it approved if no major comments are received or no member requests full committee review. This not only reduces the review period but also reduces time spent in committee.

By the time the protocol has been submitted to our IACUC for review, it has generally been reviewed by the PI's IACUC representative, a veterinarian, and the IACUC chair. Seldom do we encounter sections left blank or sections in which the PI clearly misunderstood the question. We use a protocol form similar to the one provided in Chapter 3. The form is nine pages long *before* it is completed.

We have simplified the form and attempted to make the questions clear and concise. It is available on our company's e-mail system, and it was devised so that a person can tab from one question to the next, and incorporates yes/no and check off boxes that can be answered with a single key stroke. For narrative responses, the form automatically expands so as not to waste researchers time trying to squeeze long answers into small spaces. A properly formatted form can greatly enhance researcher cooperation and aid reviewers with a clean, neat document. At a time when our company had both Macintosh and PCs, it was useful to have two sets of IACUC forms available to ensure compatibility with both platforms. Do not expect researchers to spend their valuable time reformatting forms.

Once the discussion of a protocol begins at a full committee meeting, it is impossible to predict where the discussion will lead. We have frequently erroneously predicted short meetings only to find the committee will debate a single issue for over an hour. The point is that live, face-to-face discussions usually result in more in-depth review of protocols as opposed to designating one or two members as reviewers. One person's questions or comments stimulate questions or comments from other members, frequently on issues not directly described in the protocol. Although we accuse ourselves of reinventing the wheel, we feel that it is a sign of a healthy, dynamic committee that is willing to reanalyze issues and, occasionally, reverse previous decisions based on new perspectives. The downside, of course, is that without good communication of policy changes to PIs, they will be confused and often frustrated trying to comply with IACUC decisions. Some change is good, but keep it within reason.

Most of the questions on our protocol form are straightforward, easily answered, and typically stimulate minimal discussion. Only a few seem to cause chronic problems, and the cause may be that the investigators do not understand the question. Creating clear, concise questions is essential. Maybe it is no coincidence that the questions we tend to debate the most are the ones that USDA inspectors focus on.

Listed below are sections from our IACUC protocol form that are often problematic and stimulate questions and lively debate.

Summary/Overview

This section is vital to understanding the big picture, including the scientific explanation of what the PI hopes to accomplish and why. While it is necessary to summarize *all* activities involving animals, it is not necessary to duplicate details provided elsewhere.

Justification for the Number of Animals to Be Used

USDA inspectors often want to know exactly how the number was determined and that the researchers will use the smallest number of animals possible to obtain valid results. Researchers may only be capable of making semieducated guesses, especially when working with a new, unproven animal model. If a similar study has never been performed, the variance of the data is unknown, so statistics may be of limited help. An acceptable response must include a clear, logical reason why the number was selected. If a study has never been performed by the PI but references exist, the maximum standard deviation may be used to estimate the number of animals per group. If the PI has performed the study previously, then the statistical method(s) chosen to calculate the number of animals needed should be described. This response addresses *reduction* of animal use, one of the three R's.

> *Provide a rationale for involving animals and for the appropriateness of the species.*

This question often causes the committee "heart-burn"! For a reason known only to researchers, they do not consider this to be a two-part question. They usually provide good explanations why nonanimal methods are unacceptable, but the second part is elusive. We are looking for a response that provides assurance that they are using the least sentient species possible, and that the species selected is the one that should yield the most appropriate results. Classic unacceptable responses are "mice are inexpensive" and "monkeys are closest to humans." A good response to this question demonstrates consideration of *replacement,* another of the three R's.

> *Provide a description of alternatives to potentially painful/distressful procedures that were considered and rejected. Include a description of sources used to find alternatives.*

This may be the single most important question on the protocol form. Refer to Chapter 11, The Literature Search for Alternatives. One mistake often made by investigators is to respond by discussing alternatives to conducting the whole study. USDA Policy Number 12 clearly refers to *each procedure* that may cause pain or distress. An example may be in a diabetes study that involves a partial pancreatectomy and arterial catheterization to monitor blood pressure. The discussion would need to include alternatives to the:

1. Surgery for induction of diabetes.
2. Surgical catheterization for monitoring blood pressure.
3. Potential side effects of the diabetic state.

Even though the two surgical procedures will not cause pain or distress owing to general anesthesia and postoperative analgesics, the potential for pain does exist. The appropriate response should address replacement, and possibly refinement, of each potentially painful procedure.

> Provide a description of procedures designed to assure that discomfort and pain will be limited to that which is unavoidable for the conduct of scientifically valid research.

Researchers generally provide adequate responses to this question. They may refer to the use of anesthetics and analgesics or to minimizing the intensity of noxious stimuli. Another effective method is minimizing exposure time to noxious stimuli by making it escapable or establishing endpoints at the earliest time possible to obtain valid data. This response addresses *refinement* of potentially painful or distressful procedures.

Rarely are protocols approved without revisions. If the protocol has no fundamental or major problems but requires some clarification, then the committee grants approval on condition that revisions will follow. Occasionally protocols and protocol amendments are deferred owing to the lack of sufficient information necessary to make a decision. This should be uncommon if an adequate prereview is performed. Unacceptable protocols are disapproved. After the meeting is adjourned, the committee's decisions should be promptly relayed to the PI, preferably within 24 h. Our IACUC coordinator preassigns protocol numbers so that, if approved, the number can be immediately given to the PI so that animals can be ordered as early as the next day, if necessary. The chair signs and dates the protocol as approved, assigns the appropriate USDA classification as decided by the committee, and provides a brief written justification for the classification selected. This has proven beneficial during USDA inspections. The meeting minutes always document which members were present as proof that a quorum was present. We also document that the protocol was approved, deferred, or disapproved, the required revisions, if any, the protocol title, IACUC number, the PI's name, and USDA classification.

6.6 DETAILS AND MORE DETAILS

At times, it seems that the *real* work for the IACUC administrative staff begins *after the* protocol review meetings. The AWA regulations, Section 2.31(d)(4), state that the IACUC shall notify the PIs and the research facility *in writing* of its decision to approve or withhold approval, or its decision to require revisions necessary for approval. This information is typically sent to PIs in memo form. For simple approvals without revisions, a one liner that states "Your protocol, *title,* was approved on *date."* If revisions are required, care must be exercised to accurately describe the revisions to the PI. Our IACUC coordinator transfers the exact wording from the meeting minutes to the PI's notification memo. Frequently the IACUC representative verbally informs PIs after the meeting. This allows them to make the revisions and return it to the IACUC coordinator before the meeting minutes are completed. The notification also provides the PI with the IACUC protocol number necessary to order animals. Many institutions have developed or purchased software programs linking animal purchases to the IACUC. If a computer system is not available, the IACUC coordinator provides written updates to the animal purchasing agent that lists the names of PIs who may purchase animals, protocol titles, species, and the total number of animals the PI is authorized to purchase annually under each protocol. The agent subtracts purchases from the total and notifies the IACUC when purchase requests approach or exceed the approved annual limit. Most institutions have established a mechanism to ensure that all animal purchases are IACUC-approved.

Bureaucratic glitches and human error do occur. Investigators may develop acute memory loss immediately after they receive their protocol number and forget to return their protocol with revisions requested by the IACUC. Even though it wastes time to track down investigators, we do not consider it a regulatory dilemma because technically the protocol is approved at the meeting. If the outstanding issues were of significant concern, the protocol would have been tabled for a future meeting or rejected. One week is a reasonable amount of time to expect PIs to address required revisions. We document on the signature page of the protocol form that the revisions were completed accurately. In the event that approval is withheld on a protocol, the AWA regulations state that a written statement of the reasons for its decision must be given to the PI, and the PI must be given an opportunity to respond in writing or in person. Based on this information, the IACUC may reconsider its decision. The PI may also wish to involve the IO. However, the IO does not have the authority to overturn the IACUC's decision.

IACUC may suspend ongoing activities involving animals. Reasons may include noncompliance with an IACUC approved protocol, discovery of nonapproved activities, unanticipated results that cause pain or distress to animals, inadequate training of personnel, unsafe working conditions, or issues relating to ethics. The IACUC is responsible for reviewing the circumstance with the IO, taking appropriate corrective actions, providing a written report to Animal Plant Health Inspection Services (APHIS) if involving a USDA-covered species, and for informing any federal funding agencies involved. The IACUC has several choices. It may permanently or temporarily suspend the activity or ban the PI from further animal activities, or it may allow the activities to resume after corrective actions have been reviewed. The decision is primarily influenced by the nature of the problem and the PIs response and history of infractions, if any. The IACUC's decision is final and may not be changed by the IO. Hopefully, most IACUCs will never have to make these choices.

6.7 LOOKING OVER THEIR SHOULDERS

What assurances do IACUCs have that researchers are performing their studies in complete compliance with their approved protocols? What assurance do IACUCs have that what was envisioned by the committee at the protocol review meetings is reality? No complications? No unexpected responses from the animals? Unless IACUC members go visit the laboratories periodically, it is difficult to address these questions. Although not specifically required to do so by law, it should be considered a regulatory expectation. Many institutions, including our own, have established some sort of postapproval protocol inspection or laboratory-visit process. At our institution, in addition to the IACUC Facility Inspection and Training Subcommittees, we have an Animal Studies Inspection Subcommittee, abbreviated ASIS, no pun intended. There are numerous variations on this theme. We will now describe how the ASIS operates at our institution.

The ASIS is chaired by our clinical veterinarian who is responsible for scheduling a protocol inspection approximately monthly. She typically chooses USDA Category E protocols that have the potential to cause pain or distress. Other protocols may be selected during protocol review meetings if questions are raised that cannot be answered regarding animal welfare. Inspections may focus on a specific procedure or multiple procedures conducted at different time points. They may involve multiple inspections to monitor the animal's condition, for example, with ascites production or tumor growth. Inspections are always prearranged to ensure the procedures of interest are being performed. We find it important to explain the reason for the inspection to the PI and research associates involved. Without a proper introduction, some researchers become suspicious or defensive. When we explain that the inspections are routine, they become relaxed and usually appreciate the interest in their work. They enjoy discussing the science, and the team gains a much better understanding for the entire project. The team can often provide useful suggestions that can improve both science and animal welfare.

The ASIS chair is also responsible for assembling the inspection team, usually composed of three to four IACUC members or other researchers who may have relevant expertise. More than four people tend to result in crowded conditions in most laboratories and may intimidate research associates who are performing their work. It is important not to interfere with the conduct of the study. Always be considerate of the researcher's needs.

Scheduling inspections can be difficult because they usually have to be planned several weeks in advance. Copies of the IACUC protocol and relevant amendments should be distributed before the inspection to allow team members time for review. During the inspection, team members verify that procedures are in compliance with the protocol. An exit briefing is important to verify findings and to let the researchers know what the final report will contain.

Inspection reports are written by the team member most familiar with the research, usually an IACUC representative. Reports include any relevant background information, a description of activities observed, and recommendations. Informal suggestions need not be included. If a minor protocol deviation is discovered, the report will include the requirement to submit an amendment. If the team discovers a significant problem, such as unapproved procedures that cause pain or distress to animals, the IACUC chair is immediately informed. The protocol may be suspended pending further investigation. Inspection reports frequently provide praise for individuals who perform their work with particular skill or devise unique techniques, especially if it results in reduction, replacement, or refinement of animal use. Draft reports are circulated to all team members and the PI for comments before they are finalized and sent to the IACUC chair. Final copies are also sent to the PI and the research associates named in the report. Reports are presented at IACUC meetings and filed with the original IACUC protocol.

If performed properly, researchers, IACUC members, USDA inspectors, and AAALAC site-visitors view these inspections very positively. They provide assurance that researchers are doing what they say they are doing on their IACUC-approved protocols. Questions are frequently resolved that cannot be answered while sitting in a meeting room. In particular, protocols that may sound painful or distressful on paper, oftentimes the animals demonstrate no observable effects. In a meeting, we may only surmise what the animals may feel based on experience or what we guess it would feel like in humans. Direct observation is the best method for determining the level of pain or distress. The final positive aspect of ASIS inspections is enrichment and education of IACUC members. IACUC work is usually boring. Reviewing protocols is usually boring. Discussing research with investigators and observing research as it is performed is one of the most interesting activities for IACUC members.

As in all IACUC procedures, there are many variations. Protocol inspection may not be the best terminology. Even though there is a regulatory component, a laboratory visit may convey a more collegial approach. Perhaps an IACUC has the resources to inspect the majority of approved protocols or perhaps it can only inspect protocols when problems are suspected. Inspections may be delegated to one or several individuals. Some committees may choose to do unannounced, surprise inspections. There are advantages, but there will be many times that inspectors will walk into empty laboratories. Unannounced inspections can send the message to PIs that the IACUC suspects they are doing something wrong, an attitude that certainly does little to foster a cooperative, collegial relationship. At some institutions, perhaps there is sufficient daily contact with PIs and IACUC members to assure that everyone knows what everyone else does, and there is no need to perform inspections. Every institution should develop procedures that satisfy individual needs.

6.8   ANNUAL PROTOCOL RENEWAL

Effective review of approved ongoing protocols is important for several reasons. First, it is a good method of ensuring that the PI has not changed the protocol since it was first approved. If changes occurred, then the renewal process will help ensure that the IACUC review is performed. In practice, the majority of protocol revisions are usually handled by submission of protocol amendments when the need for changes occurs.

Second, regulations, standards, and policies change and evolve over time. Often regulations do not change but interpretation does. For example, USDA Policy Number 12 on the consideration of alternatives that was issued in 1997 clarified the intent of a 1985 law. It is imperative that researchers conduct studies based on currently accepted standards.

A third reason for annual review is one of administrative practicality. It can serve as a reminder to researchers which protocols are approved under their name. If a protocol is no longer needed, it can be easily deleted at its renewal time. Removing unnecessary protocols from the list of active protocols saves time for researchers and the IACUC administrative staff.

The fourth reason should be no surprise. The AWA and PHS policy mandate it. Unfortunately, like the dissimilar requirements for composition of IACUCs described earlier in this chapter, the AWA and PHS policy differ. The AWA states that reviews shall be conducted "at appropriate intervals as determined by the IACUC, but not less than annually." PHS policy states that the IACUC shall conduct complete reviews at least once every three years. Since neither the USDA nor PHS specifies how these reviews should be conducted, institutions have developed numerous variations. The only universal requirement is that the IACUC must document the review process.

The method that the IACUC at our institution has adopted is relatively common. Several months prior to the first and second annual anniversaries of the initial approval dates, notices are sent to the PIs informing them that their protocol will expire on the anniversary date and asking them if they wish to renew or delete it. If it is to be renewed, they must describe any changes that will occur, including personnel changes. If changes affect animal use, it is brought to the committee for review. For the third anniversary, they are informed that the protocol will expire and if they need it to continue, they are required to rewrite the protocol and resubmit it for review, a process identical to the initial protocol review. This is useful for our IACUC, if for no other reason, because we revise our protocol form every one to two years to help improve regulatory compliance and to simplify the form.

There are other methods of ensuring compliance with the annual review requirement of the AWA. A time consuming method is to require complete protocol rewrites every year. Another common strategy is to require a written narrative of what was accomplished during the year along with other key questions such as updating the narrative on alternatives and asking the investigator if he/she has developed any new methods of reducing or eliminating pain or distress. There seem to be no alternatives to the PHS policy of conducting a complete review every three years.

6.9   CONCLUSION

We have described some of the many methods that IACUCs employ in carrying out the letter and spirit of AWA. What works at one institution may not work at another. It is critical to constantly reevaluate IACUC procedures and stay abreast of changes in laboratory animal care and use standards as they continue to evolve.

SOURCES AND SUGGESTED READINGS

Applied Research Ethics National Council (ARENA)/Office for Protection from Research Risks (OPRR), *Institutional Animal Care and Use Committee Guidebook,* U.S. Department of Health and Human Services, Public Health Services, NIH Publication No. 92-3415, Washington, D.C.

CFR (Code of Federal Regulations), Title 9 (Animals and Animal Products), Subchapter A (Animal Welfare), Part 2 (Regulations), Subpart C (Research Facilities), Section 2.31 [Institutional Animal Care and Use Committee (IACUC)], Office of the Federal Register, Washington, D.C., 1985.

Institute of Laboratory Animal Resources (ILAR) Committee to Revise the Guide for the Care and Use of Laboratory Animals, National Research Council, *Guide for the Care and Use of Laboratory Animals,* National Academy Press, Washington, D.C., 1996, 1.

PHS (Public Health Service), Public Health Service Policy on Humane Care and Use of Laboratory Animals, U.S. Department of Health and Human Services, Health Research Extension Act, Public Law 99-158, Washington, D.C., 1996.

USDA, *Animal Care Policies,* U.S. Department of Agriculture, Animal and Plant Health Inspection Service, Animal Care, Washington, D.C., May 1997.

7 The IACUC's Role in Education and Training

Sonja L. Wallace, A.A.S., R.V.T.

CONTENTS

The IACUC is a dynamic organization that is always adapting to changes in regulations and institutional policies—not to mention sweeping advances in science. To do so successfully, IACUCs and their institutions must train and educate staffs on the humane care and use of laboratory animals. Practical development and implementation of such a training program is usually the responsibility of the IACUC, the veterinary staff, and the laboratory animal resource staff. Many IACUCs establish a Training Subcommittee or appoint a Training Coordinator to accomplish and oversee this task.

0-8493-2580-3/99/$0.00+$.50
© 1999 by CRC Press LLC

A training program is essential to the success of an animal care and use program. Putting laws and regulations aside, perhaps the best reason to have a training program is simply because it makes good scientific sense. If animal-care personnel are trained in good, sound husbandry practices and the humane treatment of laboratory animals, the animals will be better models for research. Likewise, if investigators and research technicians have guidelines to follow for what constitutes aseptic surgery and the recommended methods for alleviating pain and distress, the resulting animal model will be much closer to a normal physiological state. The data obtained will be much more reliable because the variables will be held to a minimum. Training and education are the best way to facilitate compliance and foster a genuine regard for animal welfare issues.

And most important to the members of the IACUC, well-trained personnel will be able to prepare animal-use protocols that are well-written, follow institutional guidelines, and address the important animal welfare issues. Nothing is more gratifying to an IACUC member than acting on a protocol that they feel comfortable in approving!

This chapter will deal with the who, what, why, and how of training and where the IACUC fits in. It will discuss the federal regulations that mandate training programs in institutions—programs that cover the use of animals in teaching, testing, and research. It will also address the moral and ethical responsibility of an institution, as trustees for the animals in their care, to have such programs in place. Suggestions will be provided on how to establish an animal care and use training program and how to decide who should coordinate it. It will discuss the selection of trainers—people who are knowledgeable and are qualified to offer instruction in the various areas of animal care and use and also have the ability to speak at the level of the participants.

The chapter examines the various types of training that should be offered in-house, including lectures, seminars, workshops, wet-labs, short courses, and individualized sessions plus the availability of other resources for self-study such as access to a corporate or institutional library, setting up a laboratory animal resource and audiovisual library, and offering Internet access to the various laboratory animal science-related websites that are flooding the information highway. And it will discuss the practical implementation of a training program in this age of tight fiscal budgets and limited manpower—ways to provide training within existing resources, as well as where to look for resources that involve little expenditure of time and money. Also covered will be ways to promote attendance to training events and how to document training activities to satisfy regulatory groups.

7.1   WHY HAVE A TRAINING PROGRAM?

Both the Animal Welfare Act [Paragraph 2.32(a), (b), and (c)],[1] and the Public Health Service policy[2] stipulate that institutions are responsible for ensuring that everyone working with animals, from the animal-care staff to the persons doing the experiments, must be qualified by training and/or experience to do so. Furthermore, federal regulations designed to protect employees in the workplace require institutions to make animal handlers and users aware of the hazards and risks associated with their work.[3] Although not federally mandated, institutions should also take responsibility for training the members of their IACUC so that they are able to oversee the ethical care and use of animals in research.

7.1.1 ANIMAL-CARE PERSONNEL

According to the *Guide for the Care and Use of Laboratory Animals* (Guide), "Personnel caring for animals should be appropriately trained, and the institution should provide formal or on-the-job training to facilitate effective implementation of the program. . . ."[3] It also recommends that animal-care technicians continue to receive on-the-job training throughout their employment and they are encouraged to participate in training programs and discussions related to their work. Reference materials for consultation and self-study should be made available to the animal-care staff as well.

Changes in the field of laboratory animal science since the Animal Welfare Act was first enacted have been rapid and dramatic. Keeping animal-care personnel abreast of these changes, and continuously adjusting procedures and policies to accommodate this evolution, is of paramount importance to the animal-care program.

7.1.2 INVESTIGATORS AND TECHNICAL PERSONNEL

Institutions must evaluate the qualifications of all personnel involved in the experimental use of animals. "Investigators, technical personnel, trainees, and visiting investigators who perform animal anesthesia, surgery, or other experimental manipulations must be qualified through training or experience to accomplish these tasks in a humane and scientifically acceptable manner."[3] Because it would be impossible to have formal training programs in place for all specialized experimental manipulations, the IACUC needs assurance that a person's training and/or experience is adequate to perform the procedures described in the protocol. If not, the individual or research group must obtain appropriate training and become proficient before proceeding. This could include consulting with the attending veterinarian, bringing in outside consultants, or sending individuals to institutions where they can learn from individuals who have the necessary expertise.

IACUCs must also make investigators aware of the need to reduce and refine animal usage, as well as their obligation to search for nonanimal alternatives when designing experiments. This is usually accomplished during the protocol review process, often by incorporating these issues into the IACUC protocol form. New investigators who are unfamiliar with the protocol approval process at an institution will typically need guidance in preparing their animal care and use protocols. This is an area where training is critical.

7.1.3 ANIMAL USERS AND ASSOCIATED RISKS

The Guide advocates the establishment of formal safety programs at any institution that works with hazardous biologic, chemical, and physical agents. One function of such a program is to ensure that the staff has the training and skills necessary for the safe conduct of research. Over the years, most research institutions have established environmental health and safety programs to help comply with Occupational Safety and Health Administration (OSHA) and Environmental Protection Agency (EPA) regulations. These programs have emphasized awareness of the risks associated with blood-borne pathogens, hazardous chemicals, and radioactive materials, and how to manage hazardous waste. However, far fewer institutions have formal programs that deal specifically with the protection of the health and safety of employees who care for and use research animals. Inadequate occupational health and safety training is one of the most frequent training deficiencies cited by the Association for Assessment and Accreditation of Library Animal Care, International (AAALAC).

Instead, institutional occupational health services often rely on the IACUC or the attending veterinarian to implement training programs relating to zoonosis and animal safety. As ominous as this task may seem, training employees in the hazards and health risks associated with the care and use of research animals can, in most cases, be easily incorporated into existing training functions.

7.1.4 IACUC MEMBERS

When an institution establishes a formal training program for animal users, one group that is often overlooked is the IACUC members themselves. Anyone new to the IACUC feels apprehensive at first, particularly nonaffiliated members. The role of the IACUC is so pivotal to the research efforts of an institution that it behooves the IACUC to make provisions for training and orienting its members in the areas of federal regulations and institutional policies. Training for IACUC members is an area that is often overlooked and can include simply meeting informally with the IACUC chair, providing the individuals with a notebook of guidelines, or conducting formal orientation sessions. IACUC members should also have a basic understanding of the proper and humane care and use of animals in research so that they have sufficient knowledge to assess the appropriateness of a protocol.

At my institution, it is frequently the nonscientific and nonaffiliated members who ask the questions that prompt lively discussions at our IACUC meetings. Even though they cannot claim to be experts in animal care and use, they have sufficient knowledge to ask questions that are relevant and thought provoking.

7.2 WHO IS RESPONSIBLE FOR TRAINING?

According to the OPRR Institutional Animal Care and Use Committee Guidebook,[4] "The institution is the legally responsible entity, but the practical development and implementation of an education program will be carried out by the IACUC, the veterinary staff, and the investigators using animals." Who actually organizes the training program will depend on the size of the institution, the scope of its animal use, and the types of animal users they are attempting to train. Most institutions leave program coordination to the IACUC and/or the veterinary staff, whereas individual investigators provide specialized training.

Private industry usually has the financial resources and staffing to develop formal training programs and to make them part of the corporate directives. Academic institutions often face a larger challenge when establishing a training program because of the diverse backgrounds and needs of all the different research groups. Small biotech start-up groups must try to accomplish many tasks with a minimal staff. Workers at these organizations are already spread so thin and are wearing so many different hats that wearing the hat of trainer may assume a lower priority.

The one common denominator all these organizations share is that they are required by law to have an IACUC—therefore, it is the logical choice for overseeing the training program. Its members have a broad perspective of what specific scientific activities occur and know what the institutional needs are in regard to training programs. Their protocol review process will identify areas that need to be included in instructional programs. For example, when an investigator at a western university proposed a research project using feral armadillos, many questions in regard to the care and handling of armadillos arose during the IACUC's protocol review. It became clear that the IACUC lacked enough information about armadillos to approve the protocol and they needed more information before they could reach a consensus. This prompted a series of inquiries and consultations to educate the IACUC and the researcher's staff about how to handle and care for an animal about which relatively little was known in regard to their use in research.

At my institution, our IACUC has set up a Training Subcommittee to develop and oversee the training programs. The subcommittee is usually chaired by a member of the veterinary service staff and consists of several IACUC members and other researchers. They identify what types of training programs need to be established and how frequently they should be conducted throughout the year to accommodate new employees, student interns, and so on. They also select individuals whose background and experience, as well as their ability to train others, make them suitable instructors. In most cases, the individuals selected are veterinarians, Registered Veterinary Technicians (RVTs), laboratory animal facility managers, or research associates with specialized skills or expertise in a particular area of research.

7.3 RESOURCES

Utilizing internal resources is the most economical and easiest way to provide training. Because these individuals are already employed by the institution, training can become part of their job description or a goal toward promotion. This also assures consistency in the training program; everyone receives the same information. For example, in the blood collection technique workshops that are offered at my facility, we are fortunate to have a highly skilled metabolism group. These researchers make excellent instructors because they are the ones performing this type of work daily. They have already worked out which techniques and blood collection supplies work best for the various species and can relate well with researchers facing similar obstacles. When investigators need to learn how to place indwelling catheters, we have them work with our RTV staff; that way we know that they will incorporate good aseptic practices and effective bandaging methods so that catheters do not become a source of infection. These are just a few examples of how you can utilize people who regularly use certain skill sets in their job and can impart those skills to others.

7.4 OUTSOURCING

Smaller institutions that do not have a veterinary staff may contract with a veterinarian. Finding in-house instructors may be more problematic; outsourcing may be their best option. There are many organizations and vendors who are willing to come to your institution to give presentations or conduct training sessions. In most cases, vendors who are trying to sell a product to your organization will conduct such sessions for free. Others will speak for honoraria plus travel expenses, or will charge a registration fee for all those who attend the session. The American Association for Laboratory Animal Science (AALAS) is an excellent resource for identifying potential speakers. If an area has an active regional branch of AALAS, workshops and wet-labs may be offered at a nominal charge. If, however, outsourcing is cost-prohibitive for your institution, you might consider participating in a program sponsored by a larger institution in your town, or pool resources with several smaller institutions to distribute the costs.

For highly specialized training, such as surgical models of disease, it makes sense to bring in an outside consultant or to send individuals elsewhere for training. The Academy of Surgical Research (ASR) has a program of certification whereby applicants can become a surgical research specialist (SRS) based on the demonstration of minimal competency to perform basic aseptic survival surgery on animals.[5] The ASR Credentials Committee reviews the applicant's experience and education. Experience must be documented in the form of a surgical case log and comprehensive descriptions of surgical procedures that they have performed, including any complications that arose. A veterinarian, physician, or dentist must access competency in the operating room. Once deemed eligible, the applicant may take a certification exam. In order to maintain the SRS credential, the individual must meet continuing education requirements. There are also other organizations that offer coursework for training and certifying laboratory animal surgeons. For more information, you may contact the Academy of Surgical Research or visit their web site at www.surgicalresearch.org. Another excellent resource for information on institutions that have established their own in-house surgical training programs is the Laboratory Animal Welfare Training Exchange (LAWTE) or visit their web site at http://netvet.wustl.edu/org/lawte/homepg.htm.

For the majority of research situations, the bulk of the animal care and use training can take place in-house utilizing internal, highly skilled employees as instructors. The key to a successful training program, however, is to have an entity like the IACUC setting minimal standards and periodically reviewing the training activities for adequacy. With IACUC overseeing what type of training is taking place and who is doing it, an institution has greater control over the type of information that is being disseminated. This not only assures that an institution is meeting their regulatory obligations, but also reassures all involved that they have made their best effort possible to provide for the needs of their research animals.

7.5   WHAT SHOULD A TRAINING PROGRAM ACCOMPLISH?

What you hope to accomplish with a training program will depend upon the size and scope of the organization it serves, and the institution's philosophies. In writing *Education and Training in the Care and Use of Laboratory Animals,*[6] the authors described their intent best by stating, "The overall goals are to give personnel an overview of the scope and intent of the laws, regulations, and policies and to facilitate compliance by providing them with pertinent information and by directing them to additional skill training and resources."

At colleges and universities where there may be a high turnover of students and researchers, devoting resources to formal training in *all* areas of laboratory animal science for each animal user would be costly and time-consuming. Providing information on species and techniques that will never be used is wasteful. Instead, the emphasis would be better placed on the animal-care staff, with different research groups receiving specific training in their particular area of interest.

At smaller organizations, where investigators may have a wide variety of responsibilities, the training program needs to be much more comprehensive. For example, if an investigator at a small biotech firm is doing everything from providing the husbandry for his/her animals, to performing cardiovascular surgery on them, then the training program needs to cover those areas. It is important that the program be flexible in design to accommodate the needs of the investigators, technicians, students, and IACUC members.

Beyond fulfilling the requirements of the Animal Welfare Act and PHS policy, a training program must fit the needs of the institute, the personnel, and the animals. Overall, the training program should be used as a vehicle for heightening the animal user's awareness of the animal's needs and to encourage them to question what effect their research will have on the well-being of the animals entrusted to their care. Tables 7.1 and 7.2 provide an overview of the content and goals of an effective training program.

TABLE 7.1
Required Contents for an Institutional Training Program

Training and instruction of personnel must include guidance in several areas. Humane methods of animal maintenance and experimentation, including:

    i. The basic needs of each species of animal.
    ii. Proper handling and care for the various species of animals used by the facility.
    iii. Proper preprocedural and postprocedural care of animals.
    iv. Aseptic surgical methods and procedures.

The concept, availability, and use of research or testing methods that limit the use of animals or minimize animal distress.

Proper use of anesthetics, analgesics, and tranquilizers for any species of animal used by the facility.

Methods whereby deficiencies in animal care and treatment are reported, including deficiencies reported by any employee of the facility. No facility employee, committee member, or laboratory personnel shall be discriminated against nor be subject to any reprisal for reporting violations of regulations or standards under the [Animal Welfare] Act.

Utilization of services (e.g., National Agricultural Library, National Library of Medicine) available to provide information:

    i. On appropriate methods of animal care and use.
    ii. On alternatives to the use of live animals in research.
    iii. Unintended and unnecessary duplication of research involving animals.
    iv. The intent and requirements of the Act.

Source: USDA Regulations, 9 CFR Part 2, Subpart C, Section 2.31, *Federal Register,* August 31, 1989.

TABLE 7.2
Institutional Goals for an Animal Care and Use Training Program

Familiarize animal-care staff/investigators with state/local/federal regulations.

Familiarize animal-care staff/investigators with institutional/IACUC policies.

Introduce animal care staff/investigators to the veterinary staff, laboratory animal resource staff, and members of the IACUC; provide a tour of the facilities.

Provide information on occupational health and safety issues and zoonoses, including information on animal allergies/occupational asthma.

Provide instruction in the proper use of anesthetics, analgesics, and tranquilizers to minimize pain and distress.

Provide instruction in aseptic surgical techniques.

Provide guidelines for euthanasia.

Provide information on humane methods for the care and use of various laboratory animal species and the necessity for environmental enrichment.

Discuss alternatives to animal use and methods for reducing numbers of animals used and avoiding unnecessary duplication of studies.

7.6   HOW TO IMPLEMENT A TRAINING PROGRAM

The individuals overseeing an institutional training program need to devise a definite plan, put it in writing, and follow it through. Since the needs of the organization change from year to year, it is best to keep the plan generic in scope and update it annually. Your plan should identify course offerings and how frequently they are offered, keeping in mind that minimal regulatory requirements must be satisfied. PHS policy specifically requires that PHS-funded institutions file an Assurance of Compliance document that includes a synopsis of training and instruction offered to personnel involved with animals. Regardless of PHS funding, it is important to document all training activities to demonstrate regulatory compliance.

The types of curricula incorporated into a training program may include any of the following:

Orientations on animal care and use for new employees.
Workshops/wet-labs, lectures/seminars.
Laboratory animal technician certification classes.
Library resources and materials for self-study.
Individual training sessions/consultations.
In-house publications.

7.7   ORIENTATIONS ON ANIMAL CARE AND USE

Institutions should minimally provide all new employees, students, interns, and new IACUC members with an orientation to their animal care and use program. An orientation provides the perfect opportunity to familiarize newcomers with the organizational structure of the animal resources department, as well as to introduce them to key personnel, such as the attending veterinarian (AV), chair of the IACUC, and the manager of the laboratory animal facility. Prepackaged videos or slide presentations can be used in lieu of speakers to make more efficient use of resources for smaller audiences. Some institutions couple the orientation with a tour of the facility. Suggestions for printed materials to make available at the orientation include an organizational chart, a list of IACUC members, a map of the animal facility, and a directory of laboratory resource personnel.

An orientation session can provide a brief overview of the required contents for an institutional training program (see Table 7.1). Because it is impossible to cover each of the topics listed in a single session, the orientation should be used as a vehicle for providing information on what resources are available for further study and consultation. At my institution, we require all current employees to attend a formal orientation on laboratory animal care and use every two years to update them on changes in regulations and institutional policies. It is our way of ensuring regulators that our training of personnel is ongoing throughout their employment. Since the USDA takes a performance standards approach to evaluating training programs, the institution needs to demonstrate that their program is adequate in the context of the research performed at the institution and it meets the researcher's needs. Requiring periodic retraining is a good way to satisfy that need.

Orientations provide a forum for discussing the regulations and standards set forth by the Animal Welfare Act and PHS policy, and the means of reporting deficiencies in animal care and treatment. New employees and students, in particular, may feel uneasy about disclosing deficiencies or noncompliance issues; they need to be reassured that they will not be discriminated against or be subject to reprisal for reporting violations.

The orientation is also an appropriate time to discuss ethics and animal welfare vs. animal rights. Those who attend the orientation may be new to the world of animal research; they need to know how the institution is addressing animal welfare issues. Helping new researchers and animal care personnel develop a positive attitude toward how the facility uses animals in research will help alleviate ethical concerns that they may have about animal research in general.

Orientations are also useful for discussing the role and responsibilities of the IACUC. Unless an individual is routinely writing animal care and use protocols, they may not even be aware that an IACUC exists. This is an opportunity to educate the staff about their important function as protectors of animals used in research.

7.8 WORKSHOPS/WET-LABS

Workshops and wet-labs are particularly useful for teaching basic laboratory techniques and procedures for the various species of animals. Lecture, combined with audiovisual materials, printed handouts, and hands-on practice gives participants the knowledge and skills that enable them to perform their work. Wet-labs should be species or technique specific and enrollment should be kept small. Sessions should provide participants with an opportunity to take part in skill-building activities like animal restraint, and performing procedures such as dosing or blood collection. It is advisable to have a generic training protocol in place, with the attending veterinarian or course coordinator listed as the principle investigator, so that animals can be ordered for hands-on training sessions.

Workshops should start with a short lecture, video presentation, or demonstration to provide background information. Training videos are available from AALAS or the American College of Laboratory Animal Medicine (ACLAM). Where possible, students can practice with models such as the Koken Rat or Koken Rabbit (Koken Co., Ltd., Tokyo, Japan) before handling live animals, especially if the participants have limited or no previous animal handling experience. Also available are interactive tutorial CD-ROM programs such as *Anesthesia of Rats* (BSL Publishers, Netherlands), and *The Virtual Heart* or *The Virtual Lung* (UC Davis School of Veterinary Medicine, Davis, CA) that use computer technology to enhance the learning experience.

As mentioned earlier, IACUCs may insist that researchers attend certain workshops before they are allowed to initiate a particular animal-use protocol. For example, before allowing researchers to perform survival surgery on rodents, they could be required to attend a workshop on aseptic surgical techniques. This type of basic training helps to prevent sepsis, saving the researchers time, and keeping the numbers of animals used to a minimum.

The needs of your institution will dictate the topics that you should make available and the frequency at which they are offered. When coming up with ideas for workshops, remember that they do not necessarily have to involve the actual use of animals. Here are some suggested topics for workshops and wet-labs that can be offered:

Basic laboratory techniques in rodents, dogs, swine, nonhuman primates, rabbits, or cats.
Aseptic surgical techniques.
Surgically implanting osmotic infusion pumps in laboratory animals.
Care and maintenance of chronically instrumented animals.
Providing environmental enrichment and socialization for laboratory animals.
Anesthetic monitoring in laboratory animals.
Performing a comprehensive literature search for alternatives.
Writing animal care and protocols.
Coping with euthanasia-associated emotional stress.

7.9   LECTURES/SEMINARS

Inviting guest lecturers and speakers to give presentations is a good way to convey new technologies and advancements in laboratory animal science to the animal-care staff and researchers. Hosting outside speakers and consulting groups typically involve honorariums and travel expenses. As mentioned before, vendors often provide speakers and presentations at no charge to an institution if they are courting your business. This is particularly true of the larger laboratory animal vendors who frequently employ well-known experts in the areas of husbandry, genetics, nutrition, facility design, and laboratory animal medicine.

Seminars provide an excellent forum for discussions on occupational health risks associated with animal work. You can invite someone from your occupational health group or have the attending veterinarian give a presentation on blood-borne pathogens, zoonotic diseases, prevention of illness, prevention of acute injuries from lifting or slipping, hearing loss, first aid for animal bites, scratches, or needle-sticks, animal allergies and occupational asthma, and musculoskeletal over-use syndromes associated with animal care like repetitive motion injuries (OPRR 1992, C-5). Because the material will be pertinent to all who work with animals, conducting a formal seminar once a year and inviting all animal users to attend makes the most efficient use of available resources.

7.10 LABORATORY ANIMAL CERTIFICATION COURSES

People caring for animals must be qualified to do so. One way to accomplish this is by offering nondegree training with certification programs for laboratory animal technicians and technologists. AALAS offers a highly regarded certification program. They provide student manuals, audio–visual materials, instructional guides, and lists of reference materials to help institutions set up their own training classes in order to prepare their employees for the three levels of certification: Assistant Laboratory Animal Technician (ALAT), Laboratory Animal Technician (LAT), and Laboratory Animal Technologist (LATG).

At my institution, AALAS certification is a goal that all animal-care personnel work toward as part of their employee development. Using our own laboratory animal facility and veterinary services personnel as instructors, we offer in-house AALAS classes that are geared toward the ALAT level of certification. Classes are offered for an hour each week for 10 to 12 weeks each year. For the LAT and LATG levels of certification, employees are provided manuals for self-study and are given time during work to study in preparation for the exams.

The National Research Council's *Education and Training in the Care and Use of Laboratory Animals* is another useful guide when designing a laboratory animal certification program. It presents the information in modules with easy to follow outlines. The course content is similar to what is presented in the AALAS manuals with most of the emphasis placed on fulfilling regulatory obligations for training. The guide also has an excellent bibliography to help instructors prepare their presentation materials.

When setting up a program for laboratory animal certification, it is helpful to schedule classes well in advance and at a convenient time so work and study schedules can be adjusted to permit attendance. It is also a good idea to reserve a training or conference room that is in a convenient location and has appropriate lighting, acoustics, and audiovisual equipment to support the needs of the instructors as well as those of the students.

Instructors should be chosen on the basis of their expertise, keeping in mind that they will need to speak at the level of the participants. For example, a supervisor from the cage-washing area would make a good person to talk about sanitation in an animal facility. Alternately, you could have the attending veterinarian teach all the classes; however, we have found that students appreciate a change of pace, especially when they are getting information from the perspective of those who are responsible for a particular job. Further, the work of putting on many classes can be spread among the ranks, utilizing available resources, without overtaxing one particular person or group.

Another consideration for offering coursework for laboratory animal certification is to take advantage of the Purina Mills Laboratory Animal Care Course, the Redlands Community College Associates degree program in Laboratory Animal Science, or any of the other correspondence courses currently available for the self-study of laboratory animal science. The main drawback with these programs is that the individual has to be self-motivated and willing to spend time outside work to study and complete assignments. This approach has a better chance of success if the students are given time during work to study and have access to tutors.

7.11 MATERIALS FOR A SELF-STUDY/RESOURCE LIBRARY

If your institution has a library, you should meet with the person in charge of acquisitions to make sure that there are sufficient resources on the various subjects related to laboratory animal science. Depending on your budget, you may want to consider setting up your own library dedicated to resources for self-study. Initially include the suggested reference materials for the AALAS exams, as well as subscriptions to several scientific journals, such as the *Journal of the American Veterinary Medical Association, American Journal of Veterinary Research, Laboratory Animal Science,* and *Contemporary Topics in Laboratory Animal Science.* Examples of the types of texts to include are:

Texts on husbandry, breeding, and biology of various laboratory animal species.
Veterinary texts on health and disease.
Anatomy/physiology texts.
Texts on animal models of disease/surgical models in biomedical research.
Texts on behavior and environmental enrichment.
Texts on zoonoses and occupational health risks in animal research.
Pathology and clinical pathology references.
Texts on laboratory animal facility design and management.
Texts on biostatistics.
AALAS manuals (ALAT, LAT, LATG).
Medical Dictionary.
Physician's Desk Reference.
Veterinary formulary.
Veterinary pharmaceuticals and biologicals.
Report of the AVMA Panel on Euthanasia.
Government publications (Animal Welfare Regulations, PHS policy, Good Laboratory Practices, etc.

Texts on alternatives to animals in research.
In-house standard operating procedures or operational guidelines.
In-house IACUC guidelines.

Also include audiovisual materials like videotapes, audiotapes, CD ROMS, anatomical models, and slides. A VCR should be accessible when it is not being used so individuals can view videotapes at their leisure. Many universities and teaching facilities are producing virtual computer programs for instructing students in anatomy and physiology as an alternative to using animals in anatomy laboratories. These tutorials make excellent additions to a collection for loaning or for viewing at a computer workstation set up within a library. Computer-based training (CBT) uses active rather than passive training methods that allow people to work at both their pace and their level of comprehension. Once a CBT program is in place, it can reduce training time by up to 20 percent and increase material retention by 20 percent.[7] However, the initial setup is very time consuming. Companies like MicroMedium Inc. [www.micromedium.com, (800) 561-2098] have software available that can enable trainers to create an interactive, multimedia CBT, then distribute it, and track employee performance over Window-based networks. Computer workstations that can access the Internet provide an excellent means for personnel to explore web sites dealing with animal welfare and alternatives to animal use. Refer to Chapter 11, The Literature Search for Alternatives and Appendix 6, IACUC Resources on the Internet of Interest to IACUCs.

7.12 INDIVIDUAL TRAINING SESSIONS/CONSULTATIONS

Staff members should be identified for individual instruction and consultation. Usually, this responsibility falls upon the attending veterinarian and the RVT staff. For specific procedures or techniques, hire consultants or send individuals out for specialized training. Identify someone at your institution to field inquiries and make arrangements for individualized training so that requests do not go unanswered. If your IACUC has a Training Subcommittee, the chair is the likely choice for this role.

7.13 IN-HOUSE PUBLICATIONS/WEB SITE

Because of the regulated environment in which we work, most institutions have already written standard operating procedures (SOPs), or operational guidelines for the various tasks and duties within the laboratory animal facility. Some institutions have produced an IACUC Guide or manual that covers subjects ranging from animal procurement to permissible forms of euthanasia. These in-house publications should be made available in your resource library or can be placed electronically on an internal web site so that personnel can access the information. This IACUC Guide can be used to help satisfy some of the mandatory training requirements for an institution. The responsibility for writing this guide can be spread among the animal resources staff and IACUC members. It will have to be periodically updated to reflect revisions and policy changes.

An in-house newsletter is also an effective means of communicating with the personnel throughout the facility. It can be used to announce personnel changes, regulatory updates, new programs and services, and so on. Newsletters keep the lines of communication open between the people in animal resources and those doing research (see Appendix 6, IACUC Resources on the Internet of Interest to IACUCs).

7.14   INCENTIVES FOR TRAINING

Perhaps the biggest hurdle for any training program is encouraging the participation of researchers and animal-care personnel. Requiring attendance prior to granting protocol approval or as part of a new employee checklist is one way to guarantee compliance. If certain parts of the training program are mandatory, they should be offered at frequent intervals, convenient locations, and at times that are minimally disruptive to most work schedules. This is an area where CBT may be particularly useful because it can be done at the participant's leisure and at his or her own pace. Individuals who do not complete the training could be denied access to the animal facility or prevented from ordering research animals for experimental purposes until such training can be obtained.

For training that does not fall into the category of mandatory training, the coordinator may have to resort to more creative means of encouraging participation. If your institution has interoffice mail, e-mail, or a voice mail system, broadcast messages can be sent detailing the training activity, time, date, location, and whom to contact with questions. Make use of seminar notice boards and employee break rooms to post flyers about the training activity several weeks in advance; use attractive designs and bold colors to get attention. Notices can also be posted in newsletters or on web sites for the laboratory animal resources group. Try to spread the word in as many ways as possible to generate interest and hopefully attract an audience.

Participation in certain training activities, such as AALAS certification classes, can be linked to employee development goals. Those who consistently attend classes and demonstrate a passing score on the certification exam(s) could be rewarded with a promotion or cash bonus. If your institution's budget will not allow for monetary compensation, perhaps the person can be rewarded with extra vacation days, preferred parking, or a plaque or certificate that can be proudly displayed as a means of recognizing his/her accomplishment.

One of the best ways to encourage attendance at seminars and lectures is to simply offer refreshments. It is amazing how many participants can be drawn to events with the promise of free food! Where appropriate, you can raffle off items or give away gifts like notepads or pens and pencils embossed with the name or logo of your organization. At my institution, the environmental health and safety group gives out coffee mugs with safety messages printed on them to those who participate in hazardous material training. However you choose to encourage participation, just make sure people come away feeling it was time well spent and that their attendance was recognized.

7.15   DOCUMENTING TRAINING ACTIVITIES

It is recommended that you prepare a document describing the institutional training program to provide documentation of how the training program is being executed. At my institution, our training plan is written as one of our operational guidelines. It also appears in our AAALAC International Program Description and in our IACUC Guide.

Tracking training activities can be fairly simple. Design a generic sign-in form listing the course title, date, instructor, names of the individuals attending, and any other pertinent information, and distribute it to all instructors prior to conducting any type of orientation, workshop, seminar, or individual consultation. The training coordinator needs to make sure these forms get completed and are filed in a central location so that they can be offered as proof of training activities, if requested, during a USDA or AAALAC inspection of the facility. Alternately, you can save meeting notices or flyers and file those in your training activity file—but actual lists of attendees will have more credence and can be used to update an individual's training file. Discussing methods of documenting training activities with a USDA veterinary medical officer may also be useful. Most experts agree that providing an adequate paper trail is always advisable.

Every six months, the training coordinator should summarize the training activities and present a report to the IACUC. This is when the sign-in sheets are particularly useful because they accurately record the number of attendees.

7.16   CONCLUSION

You are now armed with some ideas on establishing a training program that meets your institution's needs while satisfying regulatory agencies. In order for the program to be successful, you will need to continue to *feed and care for it* by continuously evaluating its relevance to your current needs. Your training program should be responsive to changes in regulations and institutional policies; it must be flexible. Instructors need to be evaluated for their effectiveness and ability to train others. Individuals who have received the training should be surveyed to determine the value of the courses.

As overseers of animal care and use, the members of the IACUC have the power to change attitudes and behavior toward the use of animals in research. Through a carefully constructed training program, they can better serve the institution, its students, researchers, technicians, and, most importantly, its animals.

REFERENCES

1. Code of Federal Regulations, Title 9, Animals and Animal Products, Subchapter A, Animal Welfare, Office of the Federal Register, Washington, D.C.
2. Public Health Service, *Policy on Humane Care and Use of Laboratory Animals,* U.S. Department of Health and Human Services (PL 99-158, Health Research Extension Act, 1985), Washington, D.C. 1996.

3. National Research Council, *Guide for the Care and Use of Laboratory Animals,* from Subpart C, Section 2.31, *Federal Register,* August 31, 1989, National Academy Press, Washington, D.C., 1996.

4. National Institutes of Health/Office for Protection from Research Risks, *Institutional Animal Care and Use Committee Guidebook,* NIH Publication 92-3415, Washington, D.C., 1992.

5. Dennis, M. B., Surgical training and personnel qualifications, in *Research Animal Anesthesia, Analgesia and Surgery,* Smith, A. C. and Swindle, M. M., Eds., Greenbelt, MD, Scientists Center for Animal Welfare, 1994, 11.

6. National Research Council, *Education and Training in the Care and Use of Laboratory Animals: A Guide for Developing Institutional Programs,* National Academy Press, Washington, D.C., 1991.

7. Stark, D., Converting to computer-based training: successes, pitfalls and tips, Laboratory Animal Welfare Training Exchange, St. Louis, August 21, 1998.

8 The IACUC and Laboratory Animal Resources

Joanne R. Blum, D.V.M.

CONTENTS

8.1 INTRODUCTION

This chapter explores animal facility-related issues that require oversight by the Institutional Animal Care and Use Committee (IACUC). These issues tend to fall into

0-8493-2580-3/99/$0.00+$.50
© 1999 by CRC Press LLC

two categories: physical plant and programmatic issues. In the past, animal facility oversight concentrated on physical plant deficiencies—peeling paint, chipped floor surfaces, and similar effects of wear and tear—rather than on how the animal facility conducted its business. Recently, there has been a shift in emphasis to dealing with those policies, practices, and programs that assure animal care, animal and personnel safety, and compliance with institutional and regulatory or accrediting agency requirements. For the most part, this shift reflects a growing awareness of quality standards of physical plant development and maintenance and a high degree of compliance with regulatory requirements.

Members of IACUCs, in meeting their legal, moral, and ethical responsibilities to oversee research animal programs, must consider the need to facilitate research, assure animal welfare, and assimilate all of the publications, issues, and practices relating to the use of laboratory animals. We will endeavor to provide a brief overview of animal facility related physical plant and programmatic issues that are commonly encountered by IACUCs. In addition, suggestions will be provided on ways that IACUCs can deal with the many sources of information and topics of animal research and welfare needed to assure a knowledgeable oversight of animal facilities.

A number of internal and external references are available to IACUCs to assist them in identifying and addressing animal facility related issues. The regulations of the Animal Welfare Act (AWA) and the Public Health Service (PHS) policy, as spelled out in the Institute for Laboratory Animal Research (ILAR) publication the *Guide for the Care and Use of Laboratory Animals* (known as the Guide), require IACUCs to thoroughly evaluate physical plant and programmatic issues associated with the research animal facility a minimum of once every six months.[1, 2] Objective, *engineering-based standards* delineated in these publications are relatively easy to observe. It is a simple task, for instance, to determine that an animal is being housed in a cage that meets minimum mandated space requirements or that the environmental temperature in an animal room falls within the mandated range for that particular species. Implementation of *performance-based standards* pose more of a challenge because they rely on knowledge of individual species, state-of-the-art practices, and current and emerging technologies. In other words, a checklist approach—yes the animal is in an appropriate sized cage or no the animal is not in an appropriate sized cage—can be created to satisfy oversight of objective review or inspection points. It is more difficult to use a checklist approach to review whether or not an animal is receiving appropriate enrichment that promotes its psychological well-being. Some institutions have discarded the check list approach to animal facility inspections and have moved instead to a written narrative that not only describes observed deficiencies and provides suggested corrective actions, but also praises good practices and procedures. Care should be taken to ensure that thorough coverage of all items is made and superficial impressions, or reliance on the animal husbandry staff or laboratory animal veterinarian, are not used as the sole means of assuring compliance with physical plant standards.

This does not mean that all IACUC members must be completely familiar with all of the details listed by every applicable regulatory or accrediting agency. It would be ideal, but hardly practical, if everyone on the committee had such a thorough level of knowledge, but relying solely on the professional laboratory animal staff for guidance and expertise on animal related issues is not the answer. Even after many years in the field of laboratory animal medicine, we still have to look up specific citations—not only because we cannot memorize every word of every applicable rule or regulation, but also because rules and regulations change over time—either in content or in interpretation. It is essential, therefore, for IACUC members to be familiar with what is covered by rules and regulations, where they can be found, and who can provide expertise or assistance in understanding and implementing both the letter and the spirit of the laws and guidelines.

8.1.1 WHO GOVERNS WHAT?

There are myriad rules and regulations that govern the care and use of animals in research. At an international level, transportation of certain biological materials (e.g., cell lines or products containing animal components) and endangered or nonindigenous species of animals may be regulated by both the exporting and importing country. The U.S. Department of Agriculture (USDA) administers the AWA and the Office for Protection from Research Risks (OPRR) oversees compliance with the Public Health Service (PHS) policy and the ILAR Guide in the United States. The Association for Assessment and Accreditation of Laboratory Animal Care, International (AAALAC) also uses the Guide as a standard for voluntary evaluation of animal care and use programs. In addition, the Drug Enforcement Administration (DEA) controls the use of potentially abusive substances, including some of the anesthetics and analgesics used for animals. The Food and Drug Administration (FDA) oversees Good Laboratory Practices (GLPs) and Good Manufacturing Practices (GMPs) that may impact research conducted on animals in some facilities. Some states, California notably, also regulate the importation of nonhuman primates into the state; extend restrictions on controlled substances to drugs, such as ketamine hydrochloride, that are not currently regulated by the DEA; require registration of research facilities that are not covered by the USDA or the Office of Protection from Research Risks (OPRR); inspect facilities for worker safety and environmental infractions; and, through the Department of Fish and Game, prohibit importation of certain species of animals considered detrimental (e.g., ferrets, African-clawed frogs, etc.) except in special instances where permits may be granted.[3]

Laws at the county or city level may also require special permits for housing of certain species of research animals. Additionally, they may regulate sewer discharges, disposal of animal waste and carcasses, and the amount or type of chemical or biohazardous waste that is being stored and used in the animal facility. *It is incumbent upon IACUCs to determine which of the many regulations and guidelines apply to their institutions, familiarize themselves with the content of the applicable statutes and policies, and oversee compliance by animal care and use program participants.* They may have to enlist the help of someone, frequently a laboratory animal veterinarian, who is familiar with the regulatory mandates of a particular location. Some institutions have created research compliance positions staffed by personnel whose function is to advise the institution on applicable rules and regulations and assist in compliance oversight. Relying on doing things the same way as another biomedical research institution may not always ensure compliance with all applicable rules and regulations.

8.1.2   WHO CAN HELP?

Large institutions may have many internal resources to assist researchers and IACUCs with animal facility issues. Attending veterinarians and other IACUC members who have expertise in the use of a particular species of animal or area of research can provide insight on proper husbandry, care, and use of many laboratory animals. Librarians can provide assistance in alternative searches for replacement of whole, live animals, use of a phylogenetically lower species, reduction in numbers of animals needed or refinement of techniques (the three R's of animal research: replacement, reduction, and refinement). Computer support groups can create customized programs or assist in the acquisition of commercially available software that can organize much of the information needed by the IACUC. Computer resources can be used to record information about research animal proposals, track the numbers of animals used on particular projects (and the pain/distress category associated with that research), tabulate animal census information, and link animal medical records and diagnostic laboratory results. Subcommittees with experience or special knowledge of a particular issue or type of research can be formed from IACUC and/or non-IACUC members to provide advice to the committee. Some institutions have found it helpful to include a member of their health and safety department as a voting member or nonvoting advisor to the IACUC or, at the least, invite biosafety experts to attend relevant IACUC meetings and inspections.

Smaller institutions may not have sufficient internal resources to resolve animal facility-related questions or other issues that need to be addressed by the IACUC. In these instances, outside consultants can be solicited to provide the committee with expertise. Many institutions are willing to share their templates for everything from animal research proposal (protocol) forms to semiannual inspection forms. Much information can also be obtained from the web pages of institutions who have placed information concerning aspects of their animal care and use program on the World Wide Web. Should an investigator request a new species of animal not previously housed in the animal facility or an alternative method of housing or care, information on the proposed change can be solicited from other institutions or outside experts. Dialogues with accrediting and regulatory agencies can provide additional resources. We have had many conversations with representatives of these agencies regarding hypothetical situations and how best to approach solutions that would be acceptable to the institution as well as the agencies.

The OPRR has developed a web site (http://www.nih.gov/grants/oprr/library_ animal.htm) with a number of documents and even a tutorial that can assist IACUCs in learning what their duties and responsibilities are and how to carry them out. One of the documents that can be downloaded from this site, and then customized to the individual institution's needs, is a template for semiannual inspections of animal care and use programs and facilities. This template provides an easy step-by-step walk-through of what and how items should be reviewed during the mandated semiannual IACUC inspections. We have found this checklist particularly helpful in educating new IACUC members about the scope and framework of their responsibilities.

Another resource that is available through this web site is the *Institutional Animal Care and Use Committee Guidebook,* which was prepared by OPRR and the Applied Research Ethics National Association (ARENA). It provides a brief but informative overview of many aspects of IACUCs, including issues of documenting facility and program reviews, special considerations on the use of farm animals in biomedical research, and evaluation of animal health and husbandry.

Previous inspection reports can also be used to provide guidance to IACUC members. By reviewing past semiannual IACUC and USDA inspection reports, previously cited deficiencies can be identified and these specific areas of concern can be reviewed and evaluated. In addition, these reports may help to familiarize new IACUC members with types of issues and items that are considered, methods on how to document concerns, and other aspects related to the evaluation process.

8.2 ANIMAL FACILITY—PHYSICAL PLANT ISSUES

Animal facility-related physical plant issues are usually brought to the attention of the IACUC in two ways: when inspections occur and when renovations or new building plans are proposed.

Public Health Service (PHS) policy and AWA regulations require that IACUCs evaluate animal care and use programs (including conducting physical plant inspections) at least once every six months. Agencies or organizations such as the USDA and AAALAC, International may also conduct inspections of animal facilities and programs, and the results of their findings should be discussed at subsequent IACUC meetings. It is also prudent—although *not* a responsibility required by regulatory or accrediting agencies—to include IACUCs throughout the planning, design, and construction phases of renovating or building animal facilities. IACUC involvement in these processes can assist in addressing concerns regarding animal welfare, including adherence to mandated requirements for animal facilities and required components of survival surgical facilities for nonrodent species, are met.

Physical plant facility issues usually have more defined, quantifiable parameters than programmatic issues. IACUC members can obtain information on animal facility and other relevant issues from a variety of resources. They can obtain guidance by reading applicable federal publications that specify rules and regulations, viewing available documents and tutorials, and attending relevant meetings or workshops (such as those sponsored by OPRR, the American Association for Laboratory Animal Science, or Public Responsibility in Medicine and Research).

Educating oneself about animal facility physical plant issues, including learning how to properly conduct semiannual inspections, is rarely a top priority for most IACUC members. Many are occupied with conducting research, writing scientific reports or articles, balancing budgets, and attending meetings that are relevant to their primary job functions. However, IACUC members should not rely on only one member—usually, the laboratory animal veterinarian—to provide the expertise in how to conduct facility inspections. Nor is it feasible for all IACUC members to become experts in all phases of facility review and inspection. Institutions can assist IACUCs in gaining a working knowledge of facility and program evaluations by providing training sessions prior to inspections to familiarize IACUC members with proper inspection procedures.

Every IACUC member has the responsibility to oversee the animal care and use program at his or her institution, including the conduct of semiannual inspections of facilities, but not every institution needs to carry out this responsibility in the same way. Small institutions frequently include semiannual inspections as an agenda item during a regularly scheduled IACUC meeting. It would be best if all IACUC members tour all facilities involved in the animal care and use program, but this is not always feasible. Large institutions with multiple, decentralized animal research facilities may not only prefer to but may need to use subcommittees composed of different IACUC members to visit different animal facility sites. This divide-and-conquer approach is one practical way to handle the time-consuming IACUC task of visiting all animal facilities at least once every six months; however, caution needs to be exercised to assure that all subcommittees conduct inspections at different sites according to standardized criteria and formats. In this scenario, someone also needs to collect all necessary paperwork from different subcommittees and formulate coherent communications to be forwarded to the institutional official as well as individuals that need to know of or act on the inspection committee's findings. Ad hoc consultants may also be employed to assist in conducting semiannual inspections, but, as stated in USDA regulations, at least two IACUC members must be present.

Regardless of the approach to semiannual inspections (full committee or subcommittee), it is necessary that people conducting the inspection understand what they should look for and how they should document their findings. We are proponents of the checklist approach to most inspections and feel that the ultimate determination for evaluations should be based on actual regulatory requirements rather than subjective assessments. The following is a brief common sense overview of items that should be evaluated during animal facility inspections.

8.2.1 ANIMAL FACILITIES

Animal facilities should meet the following general conditions:

- Facilities should be structurally sound and in good repair.
- Facilities should have regularly scheduled, documented pest control programs for vermin (e.g., rodents, birds, insects, etc.).
- Facilities should provide for separation of species and isolation of sick or quarantined animals.
- Interior surfaces of animal facilities should be impervious to moisture and easily sanitizable; there should be **no** exposed, unsealed wood.
- Lighting should be sufficient for thorough cleaning and inspection.
- Emergency provisions, including availability of backup power for vital operations, should be readily available. Information on personnel to be contacted in case of emergencies should be posted in the animal facility.
- Appropriate procedures should exist for the collection, storage, and disposal of animal waste, animal carcasses, and hazardous waste.
- A program for veterinary care, including provision for emergency/weekend/holiday care, disease surveillance and control, diagnosis, and treatment, should be established and implemented under veterinary supervision.

8.2.2   ANIMAL ROOMS/CAGING

The following standards should be followed for animal rooms/caging:

- Environmental variables such as temperature, humidity, light cycles, ventilation, and noise level should be controlled and recorded. They should be appropriate for the species housed and the research project design.
- Daily observations of animals, including weekends and holidays, should be practiced and appropriately documented.
- Caging should contain animals securely and safely, protect them from other animals or extreme environmental conditions, and meet or exceed minimum regulated space requirements. Cages should be species appropriate, maintain animals in a clean and dry state, minimize scientific variables, and allow easy access to nutritious, palatable, and noncontaminated food and potable water.
- Cages and food/water receptacles should be sanitized at least once every two weeks or more often, as needed.
- Written programs and documentation of implementation should exist for the exercise of dogs and psychological enrichment of nonhuman primates.
- Animals should be properly identified, and records as to the source, dates of acquisition and disposition, and assigned project should be maintained.

8.2.3   ANIMAL SUPPORT AREAS

8.2.3.1   Cage Wash

The following sanitary/safety conditions should be practiced:

- Physical plant construction or management practices should exist to minimize contamination of clean equipment by dirty equipment.
- Quality control procedures should be in place and documented to assure adequate sanitation of caging and equipment.
- Emergency eyewash/shower stations, appropriate personal protective equipment, including, where applicable, hearing and eye protection should be available, and training on these practices provided to personnel.

8.2.3.2   Feed and Bedding Storage

The following practices for feed and bedding storage should be maintained:

- Feed and bedding should be stored so as to allow for adequate room sanitation. Prevent contamination by keeping opened bags in sealed containers. Dates of expiration (where applicable) should be clearly noted and within acceptable limits.
- Refrigeration should be provided for perishable food items.

8.2.3.3   Aseptic Surgery for Large Animals

The following procedures should be followed for aseptic surgery:

- Maintain adequate pre-, intra- and postoperative monitoring records.
- Controlled substances should be appropriately stored, with records of inventory and use, and expiration dates monitored.
- Gas cylinders should be adequately stored/secured and anesthetic waste gases scavenged.
- Aseptic procedures should be practiced for all survival surgeries.
- Functional areas for surgical support (instrument preparation), surgeon preparation, animal preparation, surgical procedures, and postoperative recovery should be physically separate or carefully separated by stringent management practices.
- Established programs for effective sanitation of facilities and sterilization of surgical instruments should be in place and monitored.
- A mechanism should be in place to document the qualifications of personnel performing surgery or anesthesia.

8.2.3.4   Rodent Surgery

The following principles apply to rodent surgery:

- Sites for rodent surgery need to be clean and not used for other purposes during surgeries. Separate, dedicated surgery rooms are not required.
- Aseptic technique and practices (e.g., sterilization of instruments, proper preparation of the surgical site, and proper attire and preparation of the surgeon including surgical gloves, etc.) should be utilized.

8.2.3.5   Personnel

The following personnel issues should be addressed:

- Administrative support areas, lockers, changing rooms, restrooms and similar facilities should be close to the animal facilities but should be located so as to minimize possible contamination.
- Personal protective equipment, work shoes, uniforms, lab coats, face masks, and gloves should be readily available.
- Programs for training personnel in proper handling and husbandry techniques should be established and documented.

When evaluations reveal concerns or deficiencies in regulatory or institutional practices or policies, they should be brought to the attention of appropriate management personnel. Reports should list the deficiency observed, relate the deficiency to a regulatory standard or institutional policy, and/or show how it is a possible threat to health or safety. By suggesting corrective actions and providing a reasonable date for corrections, the evaluators both satisfy regulatory mandates and provide guidance to the personnel who must respond to the inspection reports. Compare a report that lists "Rabbit in noncompliant cage" to a report that states "Rabbit No. 123 in Room 99A is being housed in a cage that does not meet the minimum height requirement of 14 in. as stated in the ILAR *Guide for the Care and Use of Laboratory Animals.* This minor deficiency should be corrected by June 1 by placing the rabbit in an appropriately sized cage and removing any noncompliant cages from further use." Final resolution of deficiencies should always be documented to provide assurance to inspectors that the issue was addressed. In addition, the AWA states that failure to adhere to the schedule for correction of a significant deficiency so that it remains unresolved beyond the correction date proposed by the IACUC requires written notification within 15 days to the USDA and any applicable funding federal agency.

Much debate has surrounded the issue of whether prior notification of inspection dates should be provided to personnel managing animal facilities. Our basic philosophy is that every effort should be made to have the IACUC, research staff, and husbandry personnel work together to develop and maintain a high quality animal care and use program. Therefore, we are usually in favor of prior notification of site visits because it ensures that personnel will be on hand to answer questions, interact in a positive, mutually educational fashion with the IACUC, and resolve concerns or deficiencies in a timely manner. Others feel that prior notification means that facilities will deliberately prepare for the site visit and, therefore, not be viewed under "normal operating" conditions. Obviously, each IACUC will have to address this issue, and, perhaps, modify the "prior notification" policy as the situation warrants.

It is important to document the location of all animal research facilities that are inspected by the IACUC, dates of inspections, names of inspectors, and final reports that are generated as a result of these inspections. The AWA regulations require inspection of animal housing and support facilities, including any sites where animals are maintained for greater than 12 hours. PHS policy specifies that surgical facilities and any facility where animals are maintained for greater than 24 hours be included in IACUC semiannual inspections. This AWA further requires that copies of final inspection reports be approved by a quorum of the IACUC, be signed by those IACUC members accepting the report, and include minority opinions. The reports must be sent to the institutional official. It is a good idea to document the sending and receipt of these reports in the form of a memo. Reports must be kept on file for a minimum of three years. The Annual Report to OPRR requires listing of the dates of semiannual inspections and the dates the semiannual reports were submitted to the institutional official.

Those institutions contracting animal research at remote sites need to pay particular attention to both regulatory concerns and public perceptions regarding responsibility for animal care and use at these off-site locations. Recent media stories regarding questionable animal care and use practices at some contract facilities reinforce the need for IACUCs to be involved with and develop policies concerning animal research at these locations. Responsibility for animal care, inspections, and reporting requirements should be clearly documented.

8.3   ANIMAL FACILITY—PROGRAMMATIC ISSUES

Programmatic review of animal care and use can pose unique challenges for IACUC members. Animal cage dimensions or proper member composition on the IACUC are measurable standards, but how does one measure the appropriateness of an institution's occupational health and safety program or adequacy of the program of veterinary care? Add to this dilemma the additional concerns of trying to keep abreast of current and emerging trends with regard to providing psychological enrichment to animals or housing of animals used in experiments involving recombinant DNA; even the most educated IACUC members may find their oversight responsibilities a bit overwhelming! The answer, of course, is that no one IACUC member can be an expert in all areas, and few if any committees can provide the expertise within their own membership to address all of these issues. The key is to identify those portions of the animal care and use program that should be regularly evaluated and then identify additional issues as new animal research proposals or other resources reveal topics that need to be addressed. IACUC members or non-voting advisors with expertise in relevant areas can then evaluate these concerns.

Some of the most common programmatic topics that are related to animal facilities are occupational health and safety programs, programs for adequate veterinary care, and programs of psychological enrichment for nonhuman primates and exercise for canines. Additionally, issues of research using biohazardous substances, zoonotic disease transmission from certain animal species, and research needs such as transgenic colony production can impact animal facility operation.

8.4   OCCUPATIONAL HEALTH AND SAFETY
PROGRAMS

An occupational health and safety program should be part of the overall animal care and use program and is mandated as such by the PHS policy for personnel with significant animal contact. Fortunately, there are a number of resources that facilitate establishment or review of animal facility related occupational health and safety programs. Chief among these is the National Research Council's (NRC) publication *Occupational Health and Safety in the Care and Use of Research Animals.*[4] This practical text provides a comprehensive outline on topics ranging from the development of an effective occupational health and safety program to common zoonosis of laboratory animals to ways in which institutions can address their responsibilities for providing for employee health and safety. Key elements include an assessment of employee risks for illness and injury associated with laboratory animal care and use, plus documented training on avoiding or controlling these risks; identification of physical, chemical and protocol-related hazards; emergency procedures; and a health-care service provision. Also provided in the text are references to other NRC publications dealing with handling and disposal of chemicals and infectious materials and laboratory biosafety.

Large institutions may have established occupational health and safety programs for other components of their organization that can be adapted for personnel involved in animal care and use. In these instances, the IACUC may simply function to advise the institutional official and the health service provider of its evaluation of the program. Smaller institutions may rely on the IACUC to establish and implement the occupational health and safety program. In these cases, the assistance of someone familiar with these unique programs should be requested. The attending veterinarian may be able to provide guidance on how other biomedical institutions address this issue. Occupational health departments at local medical institutions may be able to tailor a program similar to programs already in existence for other biomedical research institutions. Many biomedical research institutions are also willing to share details on their individual programs. Obviously, each institution should customize an occupational health and safety program for the needs of its own animal facility, research program, employees, visiting scientists, and/or students.

Regardless of the size of the institution conducting animal research—whether multiple animal species and hundreds of research personnel or a single species of animal and fewer than ten research personnel are involved—the following aspects of an animal facility occupational health and safety program should be examined by the IACUC:

- Does an occupational health and safety program exist, is it actively implemented, and what are the components of the program?
- Are all appropriate personnel included in the program, and what constitutes "appropriate" other than personnel working in the laboratory animal facilities, directly handling animals or animal tissues and samples?
- Does the program adequately address potential risks (e.g., provision of prophylactic immunizations such as tetanus immunization for personnel at risk for animal bites, tuberculin testing for personnel working with nonhuman primates, etc.)?
- Do procedures or policies exist for personnel protection from job-related risks (e.g., are work clothing and other forms of personal protective equipment such as face masks, gloves, and so on, provided, is there a policy on no eating/smoking/drinking in the animal facility, how are ergonomic concerns for handling animals and animal equipment addressed)?
- Is training provided to personnel on potential zoonotic risks, proper use of personal protective equipment, proper hygiene procedures, and proper procedures to follow in case of an injury or illness?

In our experience, most biomedical institutions are opting to discontinue the practice of annual physical examinations and serum banking as the backbone of their occupational health and safety program. Instead, the more practical approach of using a directed health questionnaire that is evaluated by a health professional—with referral to specialists for further evaluation on an as-needed basis—seems to better address the needs of most institutions and individuals. Use of the questionnaire, combined with practical training sessions on topics such as personal hygiene practices for personnel in contact with animals, the proper use of personal protective equipment, possible zoonotic diseases and how to prevent transmission, is a practical component of effective occupational health and safety programs. We advise all institutions to obtain input from people with expertise in various occupational health and safety-related fields. Institutions with a biosafety officer may wish to have that person serve as a voting member—or at least a nonvoting advisor—to the IACUC, so that he or she can be present at meetings and provide guidance on issues that arise during protocol review or program evaluation. Minimally, we believe it is good practice to invite biosafety officers, chemical and hazardous waste disposal managers, representatives of health care provider services, and other medical or safety personnel to tour relevant areas of the animal facility so they can gain firsthand knowledge of the environment, practices, and contact personnel in these areas. Establishing good, proactive communication and relationships between these experts and the IACUC can occur during semiannual inspections or at other times, and can prove useful to all parties concerned.

8.5 PSYCHOLOGICAL ENRICHMENT AND EXERCISE REQUIREMENTS

Years ago in the field of laboratory animal medicine, the focus was on providing safe, easily sanitizable animal housing. Enclosures had to securely contain the animal and reduce any variables that could affect the animal's health and the research data generated from that animal. Having accomplished these goals, attention moved to providing housing conducive to animal and psychological well-being as well as physical well-being. This included, but was not limited to, environmental enhancements promoting species-specific behaviors: group housing for social animals, exercise for dogs, and enrichment devices for nonhuman primates. Many of the initial endeavors to provide psychologically enriched environments for animals were governed by subjective evaluations of what people thought would be best. Scientific studies conducted over the past few years have helped to more objectively define aspects of the environment and/or practices that are most suited for animals. This remains a developing field. Biomedical research institutions housing nonhuman primates or dogs are mandated by the AWA to develop, implement, and document written plans for environment enhancement and exercise for these species. The ILAR Guide recommends that programs for animal care and use evaluate the structural environment, social environment, and animal activity patterns for the species of animals being used for research. It is becoming more common for the issue of environmental enrichment for all species—including rodents—to be questioned during AAALAC site visits. No one program is currently accepted as the standard for environmental enrichment or exercise. The intent is that research institutions—and IACUCs in particular—need to document efforts spent in developing, implementing, and evaluating improvements in the research animal's environment.

8.6 PROGRAMS FOR ADEQUATE VETERINARY MEDICAL CARE

The provision of "adequate veterinary medical care" is one of the few "must-have" requirements listed in the ILAR Guide. The term "adequate veterinary care" is also listed as a "shall have" by the AWA for research facilities. What specifically constitutes adequate veterinary care varies depending upon the size of the research institution, the species of animals used in research, the types of research projects, and the qualifications of other personnel who provide animal care and use or conduct research. Minimally, both the AWA and ILAR Guide require that research institutions employ an attending veterinarian, who will also be one of the voting members of the IACUC. Depending on the needs of the individual research institution, the veterinarian can be a full- or part-time employee or a consultant. The Guide requires that the veterinarian have appropriate training or experience in laboratory animal medicine and science or care of the species being used. When veterinarians are consultants, they must make regular site visits to the research facility and, according to the AWA, must establish a written program of veterinary care (formatted to include all the information required in APHIS Form 7002 and outlined in Policy No. 3 of the USDA *Animal Resource Guide*) that is reviewed a minimum of once a year.[5]

Regardless of whether the institution is subject to AWA, the Guide, AAALAC accreditation, or simply adhering to common practice, programs of adequate veterinary medical care are based on the following:

1. Daily observations of animals, including weekends and holidays—policies and mechanisms should be established for accurate and timely communication with the attending veterinarian regarding concerns or problems with animal health and well-being.
2. Veterinary care for animals should be available for emergencies and on weekends and holidays. Information about emergency veterinary medical care and assistance should be posted within the animal facility.
3. Programs for disease surveillance, diagnosis, prevention, and control should be in place. These should cover:
   • Procedures for evaluation of animal vendor quality.
   • Procedures for quarantine and/or acclimation of animals.
   • Policies on isolation of sick or injured animals.
   • Diagnostic resources available to assist in medical care of animals.
4. Guidance on handling of animals, appropriate analgesia and anesthesia for each species of animal, and acceptable methods of euthanasia—this should cover the assessment and alleviation of pain in animals and be in compliance with the current report of the American Veterinary Medical Association Panel on Euthanasia.
5. Provision of pre- and postprocedural care for animals. Included here are procedures for monitoring of anesthesia and analgesia, and postprocedure monitoring and care of animals.
6. Proper use of medical materials such as drugs, fluids, and suture materials. Controlled substances should be safely and securely stored and regularly inventoried. Appropriate record keeping should exist for controlled substances. Materials should be used prior to listed expiration date.
7. Oversight of surgical programs—there should be dedicated surgical facilities for nonrodent animal species. Aseptic procedures should be practiced

for all survival surgeries. Appropriate training or experience of personnel conducting procedures should be provided. There should be procedures for the proper storage, use, and scavenging (if needed) of anesthetics. Effective sterilization of surgical instruments should be monitored. Pre-, intra-, and postoperative monitoring and care of animals should be documented.

A veteran of numerous regulatory inspections and accrediting or funding agency site visits knows the value of the maxim "If it isn't written down, it can't be verified/doesn't exist/wasn't done." Therefore, though you might invoke the ire of those who believe that records in animal facilities should be kept to a minimum, you should always **document, document, document** when it comes to the provision of veterinary medical care.

8.7   OTHER PROGRAMMATIC ISSUES

IACUCs need to customize and perhaps even extend programmatic reviews to those special issues that apply to their particular research institutions. Research projects may call for the use of radioactive isotopes or the use of infectious agents in research animals. The use of such hazardous materials entails further regulatory considerations at the institutional, local, state, and, in some instances, the federal level. Depending upon the species of animals used, IACUCs may need to consider the potential for zoonotic disease transmission from certain species of animals when evaluating the training, occupational health and safety, and physical plant components of the animal care and use program. Specialized research such as the use of lasers or creation of transgenic rodent breeding colonies calls for additional institutional oversight to assure the safety of personnel and the success of the research programs. New programmatic issues identified during protocol review or semiannual inspections will trigger the need to broaden the understanding and scope of responsibility for the IACUC. And, finally, IACUCs should be involved in disaster plans.

8.8   CONCLUSION

IACUCs are faced with a number of broad and sometimes complex physical plant and programmatic issues related to animal facilities. Notwithstanding the complexity and occasional confusion surrounding these issues, it is the responsibility of IACUCs to provide thoughtful institutional oversight of animal facilities and related animal programs. It is unrealistic to believe that all IACUCs can include voting members with expertise in all of the areas that need discernment. However, the judicious use of internal resources (members of other units within the institution who can serve as advisors) and/or external resources (consultants, members of regulatory agencies, etc.) can broaden the capabilities of the committee and assist in addressing many issues facing IACUCs today and in the future. The task may seem overwhelming at times, but it is possible, with dedicated effort, to achieve comprehensive, effective and rational oversight of animal facilities and programs.

REFERENCES

1. Code of Federal Regulations, Title 9 (Animals and Animal Products), Chapter 1, Subchapter A (Animal Welfare).
2. *Guide for the Care and Use of Laboratory Animals,* Institute of Laboratory Animal Resources, National Research Council, National Academy Press, Washington, D.C., 1996.
3. State Laws Concerning the Use of Laboratory Animals in Research, National Association for Biomedical Research, 818 Connecticut Avenue, NW, Suite 303, Washington, D.C., 1991.
4. *Occupational Health and Safety in the Care and Use of Research Animals,* National Research Council, National Academy Press, Washington, D.C., 1997.
5. USDA Animal Care Policies, *Animal Care Resource Guide,* May 1997.

SUGGESTED READING

ANIMAL FACILITY DESIGN

Approaches to the Design and Development of Cost-Effective Laboratory Animal Facilities, Canadian Council on Animal Care (CCAC) proceedings, Ottawa, ON, Canada, 1993.
Comfortable Quarters for Laboratory Animals, 8th ed., Animal Welfare Institute, Washington, D.C., 1997.
Handbook of Facilities Planning, Vol. 2, *Laboratory Animal Facilities,* Ruys, T., Ed., Van Nostrand Reinhold, New York, 1991.

ENRICHMENT

Bloomsmith, M. A., Brent, L. Y., and Schapiro, S. J., Guidelines for developing and managing an environmental enrichment program for nonhuman primates, *Lab. Anim. Sci.,* 41, 372, 1991.
Psychological Well-Being of Nonhuman Primates, National Research Council, National Academy Press, Washington, D.C., 1996.

GENERAL

White, G. L., Perry, M. A., and Kosanke, S. D., A comprehensive health science center educational program for animal care and use, *Lab. Animal,* 20(7), 47, 1991.
Berry, D. J., Reference Materials for Members of Animal Care and Use Committees, USDA, National Agricultural Library (AWIC Series No. 10), Beltsville, MD, 1991.
Engler, K. P., Reference Materials for Non-Affiliated Members of Animal Care and Use Committees, SDA, National Agricultural Library (Special Reference Brief 89-08), Beltsville, MD, 1989.
Gordon, B., Unique problems of animal care and use in small institutions, *Lab. Anim. Sci.,* 37(Special Issue), 127, 1987.

OCCUPATIONAL HEALTH AND SAFETY

Bowman, P. N., A flexible occupational health and safety program for laboratory animal care and use programs, *AALAS Bull.,* 30(6), 15, 1991.
Soave, O. and Brand, C. D., Employer responsibility for employee health in the animal environment, *Lab. Animal,* 20(2), 41, 1991.
Richmond, J. Y., Hazard reduction in animal research facilities, *Lab. Animal,* 20(2), 23, 1991.

9 The Role of the IACUC in Assessing and Managing Pain and Distress in Research Animals

Sally K. Wixson, V.M.D., M.S.

CONTENTS

0-8493-2580-3/99/$0.00+$.50
© 1999 by CRC Press LLC

9.1   INTRODUCTION

One of the most crucial responsibilities of an IACUC is to make certain that pain and distress is minimized in research animals. Both the Federal Animal Welfare Act (CFR, Title 9, Subchapter A, 1985) and PHS Policy (Public Health Service, 1986) are quite clear in charging the committee with a review of research proposals (protocols) to justify and limit pain and distress in animal subjects of research studies. This chapter addresses issues that are of primary importance in determining whether or not painful procedures will be a component of a research protocol and, if so, offer strategies to minimize their impact upon the animal(s). Each institution and IACUC, depending upon its particular nature of research, teaching, and testing, will have different issues relative to pain and distress to consider: toxicology, cancer chemotherapeutics, creation and testing of biomedical devices, infectious disease models, burn therapies, and arthritis models, to name a few.

A common benchmark for evaluation of potentially distressful research methods is that if a procedure is deemed to be painful in humans, it should be assumed that it will be painful in animals. In some cases, decisions on what we anthropomorphically believe to be painful procedures are fairly clear cut. Intracranial surgery is considered to be exquisitely painful in humans, therefore, it should be assumed to be markedly painful in animals. Other experimental manipulations are not as clear-cut. Should we consider laparotomies to be painful in animals even though many of them postoperatively appear to be active, ambulating, eat, and even breed as if "nothing had happened?" In the latter situations, it becomes more difficult for the IACUC to justify requirements for protocol refinement or inclusion of analgesic therapy, particularly when the PI is concerned that these design changes may compromise the scientific integrity of the studies. Later in this chapter, we will discuss mechanisms to recognize pain and distress in laboratory animals and the role of pilot studies and IACUC subcommittee observation of procedures as a possible mechanism to evaluate whether or not animals are in pain or distress during or following experimental manipulations. When animals in pain or distress are clearly and unambiguously identified, strategies will be presented to pharmacologically (by use of analgesic drugs) and/or nonpharmacologically (bandages, special husbandry, diets, and enrichment) control and limit their discomfort. When all of the previously mentioned methods to limit pain and/or distress fail, it is appropriate for the committee to be prepared with endpoints to terminate the experiment. The bottom line is that there is almost always *something* that an IACUC can do to refine protocols to minimize both the intensity and duration of pain and/or distress in animals.

9.2   JUSTIFICATION FOR PAINFUL PROCEDURES
IN ANIMALS

An empirical decision that each IACUC must face when addressing protocols that include a component that may potentially impart pain and/or distress to research animals is whether or not animals should ethically be subjected to pain that humans would not willingly endure. Many fields of scientific endeavor involve quests to discover therapies for diseases that cause pronounced disability, dysfunction, and distress in humans. In plain language, humans are afflicted with some pretty awful maladies that may lead to a dismal quality of life, and many of us in the biomedical research business are trying to find ways to treat and cure these diseases. Therefore, is it not likely that animal models for these disease scenarios would also *a priori* require a similar degree of functional, physiological, and sensatory abnormality? Is it ethical to create genetically-altered animals that will, by definition, suffer all the afflictions and maladies of their human disease counterpart? What about pain research per se? Is it ethical to conduct this type of research on animals, knowing that you must in some way create pain in an animal to ultimately benefit humans in pain? Are there any scientific disciplines that simply should not incorporate *in vivo* study models?

Each institution, its administration, and its scientists must wrestle with this dilemma. In the author's opinion, it is not the role of the IACUC or attending veterinarian to dictate what fields of study or models that can/cannot be performed at the institution, rather it is the job of the IACUC and veterinarians to advise and counsel the PI as to how each model can be refined to perform the research within a highly ethical, scientifically meaningful, and humane framework. In this context, it is within the charge of the IACUC to justify the use of potentially painful procedures in laboratory animals if certain provisions and safeguards are clearly and unequivocally put into effect to eliminate or at least minimize any unpleasant stimulation. This may require the attending veterinarian or designated reviewer to become familiar with literature in the field relative to this protocol and to become familiar with what methods are/are not currently in use by other well-respected scientists to minimize the use of painful procedures. It is important to remember that even though the PI is highly knowledgeable about the scientific aspects of the study, they may not be aware of newer methods or technological advances that would be less stressful on the animals, and thus more acceptable to the IACUC. A thorough alternatives search can really be beneficial in this aspect of protocol review. Techniques to complete a productive alternative search are presented elsewhere in this text.

Although ample literature is available to justify the scientific value and to assist IACUCs and scientists in devising safe formats for the conduct of gene therapy and the creation of genetically-altered animals (Feldman and Hoyt, 1994; Cornetta, 1992; Hubbs, 1997), little has been written on the ethical aspects of debilitation and inferred distress in these models. IACUC members should, however, be aware that guidelines do exist for the ethical conduct of pain research in animals (Zimmerman, 1983). It is important for IACUCs to become familiar with the available literature, particularly in regard to suggestions for the humane support of these challenging models, and to develop their own guidelines when presented with novel models requiring intensive supportive care. Finally, there comes a point in a number of research studies in which further pain and suffering by the animal is unjustified, no matter how noble the cause. It is the IACUCs role to recognize when this point has come and end the research trial at this time.

9.3 ANIMAL-USE APPLICATION (PROTOCOL) FORMAT

Each IACUC usually develops its own unique animal-use application (will be referred to as protocol throughout this chapter) format that facilitates the review process. Along with the standard questions relating to the species to be used, justification of animal numbers, location where the research will be performed, and skill of the research staff, the committee must develop mechanisms to facilitate a dialog with the PI regarding additional issues relative to pain, distress, and suffering. These include a discussion of experimental methods, including anesthetic and analgesic usage, compound administration, surgical techniques, food and water deprivation, prolonged restraint, study endpoints, and methods of euthanasia. The protocol format must be generated so as to extract honest, articulate, yet comprehensive, responses from the PI to all of these questions in order for a meaningful IACUC review to take place. In other words, the committee needs to understand what the PI is proposing to do to the animals, how the study will be done, by whom, and how the study will end. Only then can a dialog begin on assessing and, if necessary, refining, reducing, or replacing painful methodologies. Frequently, institutional protocol forms offer a series of checklists to extract information of this nature; this is a helpful mechanism to assure that the PI completes each and every item and no crucial responses are left unanswered. Often, it is useful to include sample responses, such as "postoperative analgesia will be provided using morphine at a dosage of. . . ." Standardly, the PI is also asked to predict if more than momentary pain or suffering will be imparted to the animals and, if so, justify that alternatives to the painful procedures do not exist. This section of the protocol review is addressed elsewhere in Chapter 11, The Literature Search for Alternatives.

9.4 PAIN CLASSIFICATION

For species covered by the Federal Animal Welfare Act (CFR, Title 9, Subchapter A, 1985), animal numbers should be listed within the protocol by pain classification. Totals for institutional animal use in all protocols under each category during the government calendar year are then included in the institution's annual report to the USDA. Refer to The Annual Report of Research Facility, APHIS Form 7023. Any animal use classified as category E (unrelieved pain and suffering) must be justified by a written narrative on the Annual Report to the USDA. At the time that the PI writes and the IACUC reviews a protocol, this assessment comes down to an educated best guess, which is certainly fortified by previous experience with the model by the PI and committee members. When the PI is proposing the use of new animal models or will be administering substances with unknown consequences (e.g., toxicity studies), the protocol's designated pain classification may require amendment (either upgrading or downgrading of one or more groups in the experiment) after the study is completed. Indeed, it is often a reasonable and beneficial format for the IACUC to approve a protocol with a certain pain classification and request the PI to report back to them during or after the experimental trials to communicate whether the animals seemed to be in greater/lesser pain and distress than was originally antic-ipated. If a formal change in the number of animals in each pain classification scheme for this protocol is warranted, the protocol can be amended at this time. It is also important for the committee to consider the pain classification that is appropriate for the control groups. In some fields of scientific study, such as preclinical drug trials, the control group of animals may markedly differ in condition from the animals in the experimental groups that get various dosages of the compound being investigated. For this reason, the pain classification level may differ.

It is in the best interests of the animals, the PI, and the institution to devote suf-ficient effort to address this aspect of the protocol and feel comfortable with defend-ing the pain categorization assigned to the study. Few institutions and PI's relish making a public acknowledgement of category E work (the reader should remember that annual reports are available to the public by way of a Freedom of Information Act request). An assignment of pain classified as category E may, in fact, serve as an incentive to the PI to further refine the experimental methodologies to qualify the study for a less intense pain categorization level.

9.5   REVIEW POLICIES

Once the protocol is submitted, who should review it relative to issues of managing pain in research animals? The PHS policy (Public Health Service, 1986) and Federal Animal Welfare Act (CFR, Title 9, Subchapter A, 1985) define the committee com-position such that expertise to evaluate a protocol's inclusion of painful methods usu-ally exists within the local committee. Often, however, the committee review is substructured such that a designated reviewer, or subcommittee reviews the protocol in its entirety and suggests action to the full committee, with the understanding that any member may request a full committee review of any specific protocol, if he or she feels it is so warranted. In some cases, external consultants with special expertise in scientific endeavors may be advisable so that less common but complex experi-mental methods can be evaluated, including their potential to be stressful or painful to the animals.

Specific questions that relate to pain or distress and suffering are as follows:

- Species specific pain sensitivities/resistance intensity.
- Duration and frequency (chronicity) of experimental manipulations, in gen-eral; a manipulation that is not particularly painful when performed alone may become quite stressful to the animal when repetitively performed (e.g., multiple blood samplings in one day or multiple periods of restraint in a day).
- Intensity, duration, and frequency (chronicity) of overtly painful stimuli.
- Recognition of pain/distress/suffering in the research animals.
- Level of consciousness required to feel pain.
- Methods that will be employed to minimize pain and distress (such as train-ing the animals to restraint, specialized caging, appropriate methods of anesthesia, aseptic surgical technique, postoperative care, pharmacologic, and nonpharmacologic management of pain).
- Recognition of effective analgesia in the research animals.

- Intra- and post-procedural observation and recordkeeping to assess the level of comfort/discomfort in the study animals and trigger notification of appropriate personnel to take either therapeutic action or suggest euthanasia.
- Experimental endpoints (i.e., will death be an endpoint of the study or will the animals recover and return to normal or be euthanized at the termination of the study?).
- Experimental mortality—is it possible that the use of analgesics will decrease mortality in a study?
- Feasibility of pilot studies to evaluate and possibly further refine the model before approval of the definitive study.

Several of these topics will be discussed in greater depth later in this chapter.

9.6   SPECIES SPECIFIC PAIN SENSITIVITIES/RESISTANCE

Pain is a complex sensory and emotional experience, and it is probably an oversimplification to say that no two members of the same species experience and interpret the same noxious stimuli in the same way. This has historically made assessment of individual variations in pain sensitivity almost impossible in companion and research animals, particularly because they cannot verbalize the intensity of their pain experience. Lack of recognition of individual variations in pain sensitivity among and within various veterinary species has resulted in herd generalizations for analgesic therapy, such that all animals of one species are usually predicted to exhibit the same magnitude and duration of response to treatment. These generalizations have often lead to a disappointing and frustrating lack of clinical efficacy when using analgesic drugs.

Rodents have historically shown tremendous variability in responses to painful stimulation and analgesic therapy without adequate scientific rationale. Recently, however, the use of transgenic and gene targeting technology has identified rodent strains showing a strain divergence in sensitivity to experimental as well as clinically relevant pain (Mogil et al., 1995, 1996). Gene(s) have also been identified that encode for certain classes of murine opioid receptors. Substrain divergence in pain sensitivity has also been identified between animals obtained from different rodent vendors. As additional information in this area becomes available on rodent and nonrodent species, it will be useful for IACUCs to recognize these strain and species differences when reviewing protocols with a painful component and to tailor any recommendations for analgesic therapy to the particular sensitivities/resistance characteristic of that strain.

9.7   PHYSIOLOGIC CAUSE(S) OF PAIN

It is beyond the scope of this chapter to discuss the physiology of pain, and the reader is referred to several excellent reviews of the topic (Danneman, 1997; National Research Council, 1992). Suffice it to say that pain is caused by many different inciting events, and the IACUC members should focus their review and any suggestions for amelioration of pain on *methods that will most appropriately address and relieve that particularly painful stimuli.* For example, poor surgical technique may lead to infection, abscessation, and incomplete wound healing. There is little doubt that the animals are uncomfortable during these events. Treatment with an opioid analgesic should offer the animal some relief, however, the actual inciting cause of the pain is the complications of the surgery and corrective actions such as draining the abscess, reconstructive surgery to close the wound, and so on, will in the long term be most beneficial to the animals. In another example, inflammatory pain can be more effectively treated with nonsteroidal antiinflammatory drugs that decrease the cellular mediators of the immune response than with application of repetitive electrical stimuli, the latter being an effective method to manage neuropathic pain. For these reasons, the IACUC best serves its function when efforts are made to understand the source of the pain and/or distress and devise strategies to mitigate pain at that level.

9.8   INTENSITY, DURATION, AND FREQUENCY OF PAINFUL/DISTRESSFUL STIMULATION

Pain can be acute (momentary) or chronic (lasting days to weeks or even months). Experimental methods can also impart noxious stimuli one time or repetitively to the animals. It is important for the IACUC to recognize the temporal spacing and intensity of the painful manipulation(s) because this characterization will strongly influence the method(s) chosen for treatment. For example, acute, severe pain is best treated in animals using a potent analgesic drug (e.g., morphine), while chronic, dull pain is more likely to be treated with other analgesic drug classes (e.g., NSAIDS, acetaminophen, or mixed agonist–antagonists). It is unlikely, however, that a pure opioid agonist will be effective for management of long-term, chronic pain owing to development of pharmacologic tolerance. The IACUC can best serve its mission when its members recognize that all pain is not alike, and time and efforts spent to characterize its cause, intensity, and duration will be of immeasurable assistance in devising strategies for pain management.

It is also important for the IACUC to examine the overall scope and summation of experimental procedures that each animal must endure. Any of us who have been hospitalized can recall the overall level of fatigue, debilitation, and stress imparted by the sum total of the experience in addition to the memories of short duration overtly painful procedures. Such may also be the case with laboratory animals in that some proposed studies may be just too busy (i.e., too many time points in a pharmacokinetic study or too many grid shocks in a behavioral experiment) and the resultant stress becomes too great on the animals to be justifiable. In these cases, it is also the role of the IACUC to work with the PI to refine the study so that a suitable number of data points are obtained within a framework that is "do-able" and humanely acceptable. In situations of this nature, it may be useful and appropriate for the committee to remind the PI that stress, in its own right, may be just as difficult, if not more difficult, than overt pain to recognize and alleviate in a research setting. Just like pain, stress and distress may also introduce significant variability that will adversely confound the scientific benefits to be derived from the study.

9.9   RECOGNITION OF PAIN
IN LABORATORY ANIMALS

Guidelines for recognition of pain in the various species of animals used in biomedical research, teaching, and testing appear elsewhere and are beyond the scope of this chapter (Danneman, 1997; Morton and Griffith, 1984). In general, it is important for animal-care personnel, in particular, to be observant and aware of the normal behavior of the animals before any experimental manipulation occurs because it is the signs of deviation from normal that are the most common and reliable signal of pain perception in animals. Although species diversity in overt signs of pain exists, symptoms such as dysfunction, vocalization (particularly when an affected limb is moved), hunched posture, abdominal guarding, inability to rest and lie in recumbency, and aggression in a normally placid animal are all usually considered to be behavioral hallmarks of acute discomfort. Physiological signs of acute pain include rises in heart rate, blood pressure, and respiration. Chronic discomfort/pain in animals is much more difficult to assess and requires a more dedicated and objective assessment of several parameters such as weight loss, food and water consumption, general appearance and lack of self-grooming, breeding performance, and cage space utilization (the latter as a measure of activity). Methods have been developed to produce a pain scoring scheme for evaluating behavioral and attitudinal signs of pain perception in animals in which points are assigned to each parameter, such as posturing, and a cumulative score determined for each animal. Based on these point totals, decision on protocol modification, including analgesic therapy, can be made (Morton and Griffith, 1984). The task of the IACUC is to educate all concerned with the care and use of the animals on a particular protocol (i.e., the PI, research, and animal-care staffs) to observe the animals before and throughout the study to detect animals that may be in pain and to set the chain of events in motion to deal with it.

9.10   DO UNCONSCIOUS ANIMALS FEEL PAIN?

It is not uncommon for an investigator to tell the IACUC that their experimental animals do not need analgesic therapy because they are unconscious and thus unaware of painful stimuli or the painful/distressful sequelae of experimental manipulations. It has become accepted practice throughout the realm of biomedical research over the past century to prohibit the use of muscle relaxants or curariform drugs in unanesthetized animals. It is clear from the human literature and from physiologic monitoring of animals that drugs of this nature **do not** dull perception so that the subject is well aware of all sensations but cannot respond to escape the painful stimuli. Less clear is what level of analgesia, if any, is required for animals that appear to be unconscious and unaware of self and the environment. It is not uncommon for circumstances of this nature to occur in animal models used in infectious disease, sepsis, burn, dose range toxicity, and cardiophysiologic and neurophysiologic studies. In these protocols, the animals appear to be comatose and frequently advance to a moribund state. Furthermore, death has historically been an endpoint for many of these models. Should the IACUC require analgesic therapy for these animals? Accounts appear in the human literature of patients who have miraculously survived catastrophic diseases and/or trauma, and subsequently recount their feelings of marked distress and discomfort and vivid perception of noxious stimuli, yet to all accounts of observation by the medical personnel and family members they were totally and completely unconscious and nonresponsive to their surroundings (Lawrence, 1995; Schnaper, 1975). From the IACUCs standpoint, the necessity/frivolity of analgesic therapy in these models is further complicated by the historic absence of attempts to mitigate pain in study animals. As such, no benchmarks exist for validity of the studies using an analgesic format.

It is very hard for the PI, veterinary staff, or technicians to determine consciousness or unconsciousness in an animal. Aside from physiologic monitoring of changes in heart rate, blood pressure, respiratory depth and rate, and EEG patterns that can be indicative of noxious stimulus perception, there is no absolute indication of consciousness in animals. Arguably, by the time the animal becomes comatose we have lost the window when we could have intervened and made the animal more comfortable. To this end, it seems most prudent to the author that the IACUC should be most attentive in the observation of the animals while they are in a declining state of health, that is, before they become unconscious, and debate whether or not analgesic therapy would have been beneficial at the earlier stages in the animal's demise. This format is not possible with all of the models named previously, particularly those in which the altered state of consciousness is an immediate sequelae to nonsurvival surgical manipulation of the animals (e.g., spinal cord transection models). In the latter case, the dilemma frequently surrounds whether or not to terminate anesthesia while continuing data recording in a brain dead animal rather than whether or not analgesia per se is indicated.

9.11 METHODS TO MINIMIZE PAIN AND DISTRESS

9.11.1 TISSUE HANDLING, HEMOSTASIS, AND ASEPTIC SURGICAL TECHNIQUE

When performing survival surgery, postoperative pain can be greatly minimized by use of gentle tissue handling, prompt attention to blood loss, and incorporation of aseptic surgical technique. When the preceding principles are followed, there will be minimal postoperative infection, swelling, or inflammation (which are all painful events) owing to tissue destruction and wound contamination. There are many references and guidelines available in the literature as well as on the World Wide Web (home page of the comparative medicine department of many academic research institutions) that provide a format for development of institutional standards for aseptic surgical technique. It is well within the IACUCs charge to provide institutional training on these aspects of good surgical technique to minimize the animal's postoperative discomfort. The committee should also be aware that aseptic surgical technique is required for survival surgery by the Federal Animal Welfare Act (CFR, Title 9, Subchapter A, 1985) and the *Guide for the Care and Use of Laboratory Animals* (Institute of Laboratory Animal Resources, 1996).

9.11.2   NONPHARMACOLOGIC PAIN AND STRESS MANAGEMENT

Nonpharmacologic strategies to minimize pain and distress during and after experimental studies should also be considered by committee members during protocol review. It is important to recognize that analgesic drugs are not the only methods available to provide pain relief in research animals. Although acute, high intensity pain almost always requires the use of potent analgesics (usually opioids), nonpharmacologic methods such as bandaging, the use of splints and Elizabethan collars to minimize self-trauma, environmental enrichment to distract the animal, provisions of specialized diets and treats, and specialized housing all can be effective strategies to limit discomfort and distress, particularly when the pain is categorized as chronic and of low intensity. The aforementioned nonpharmacologic methods can also be of benefit when the animals are not necessarily judged to be in pain per se but rather are distressed (physical or mental anguish or suffering) by the intensity of the experimental design. Even in situations wherein the PI does not permit the use of anxiolytic drugs (e.g., sedatives and tranquilizers) to promote a calmer and less agitated animal, suggestions for alternative caging, environmental enrichment, and so on, are often well-accepted. The take-home message to the IACUC members in this regard is that something can almost always be done to benefit the animals, even when the PI can scientifically defend the deletion of analgesics and/or tranquilizers from the protocol.

9.11.3   ANESTHETIC AND ANALGESIC THERAPY

Anesthesia is a necessary component of many research manipulations that are performed on animals. It is beyond the scope of this chapter to present detailed discussion of appropriate drugs and delivery equipment to provide anesthesia for the diverse species of animals used in biomedical research. It is the responsibility of the IACUC, however, to perform a detailed protocol review such that the committee is assured that humane and scientifically acceptable methods are incorporated into the study that will make the animal(s) unaware of the procedures being done to them. Otherwise, inevitable pain and distress will occur. It is also the task of the IACUC to have among its membership expertise to judge whether or not the protocol contains anesthetic methods and delivery techniques that are safe and effective in that particular sex, age, and species of laboratory animals. Many IACUCs will provide to the PI appropriate institutional guidelines or references to detail the pharmacologic effects as well as suggested drugs and delivery methods for use on various species. The reader is referred to several excellent and comprehensive texts that specialize in anesthesia of laboratory animals (Kohn, et al., 1997; Flecknell, 1996).

   In the past, it was often argued that analgesic therapy was contraindicated for research animals because any drugs administered would impose additional variables over and above the hypothesis being studied. Recent studies, however, have shown that unrelieved pain, in itself, may profoundly alter physiological responses in research animals. For example, Liebeskind (1991) has shown that pain and stress can inhibit immune function and a tumor's metastatic growth in rats. In humans, recent studies also indicate that effective pain management can decrease surgical morbidity and mortality, see Liebeskind (1991). Thus, it is both scientifically and ethically rational to design protocols to effectively relieve pain in research animals.

There are many drugs currently marketed that are reportedly efficacious for relief of pain in animals. The major drugs available may be classified as opioid agonist, opioid agonist/antagonists, alpha$_2$ agonist, and antiinflammatory agents. The latter group contains a diverse spectrum of compounds including corticosteroids and the nonsteroidal antiinflammatory agents (NSAIDS). Other classes of drugs such as antihistamines and tricylic antidepressants have been shown to possess some analgesic activity but are, in general, clinically inferior to the opioid agents. Additionally, local anesthetics are available and may be useful to obtund localized pain when systemic therapy is not needed or would be contraindicated in a research study. It is beyond the scope of the chapter to present a comprehensive discussion of the pharmacology of each available analgesic agent and the reader is referred elsewhere for this information (Heavner, 1997). In addition to the IACUCs charge to discern whether or not a research protocol contains painful and stressful methods and suggest strategies to minimize discomfort to the animals, it is also within the committee's responsibilities to evaluate any analgesic therapies that are proposed. Analgesic drugs should be chosen based on their pharmacologic appropriateness for the study being performed and their track record in the species being used. The committee should not be misled by the mistaken theory that if a painkilling drug (and dosage) works in a human, it should surely be similarly effective in animals as well. Much diversity exists within the animal kingdom regarding the metabolism and sensitivity of its members to the various analgesic drug classes. The committee must also carefully evaluate the frequency and method of drug delivery. Currently, almost all available analgesics and the potent agents, in particular, are best administered parenterally (by injection). Albeit that research personnel are often not available to administer drug therapies around the clock, parenteral analgesic drug administration, usually at intervals of every 4 to 8 h, remains the gold standard of analgesic management in animals. Alternative delivery methods (e.g., oral, transcutaneous, or other sustained release methods) should be measured against these standards until formulations and technologies are validated that clearly indicate the production of safe and effective therapeutic drug levels in animals. The PI and IACUC should review each protocol carefully to assure that a best fit for the analgesic drug(s), dosages, route of administration, sex, age, and duration of effect for that particular species of laboratory animal is chosen. The reader is referred to several excellent and comprehensive texts for discussion of analgesic drug guidelines for use in laboratory animals (Flecknell, 1996; Kohn, et al. 1997).

9.12   CAN RELIEF OF PAIN INFLUENCE EXPERIMENTAL MORTALITY?

Sooner or later, an IACUC will be faced with the support of a research protocol that produces high (e.g., greater than 50 percent) experimental mortality. At times, mortality is influenced by the complexity of the experimental procedures (often surgical manipulations) and all efforts to eliminate any other possible causes of morbidity and mortality (e.g., postoperative infection or failure of implanted devices) do not yield greater overall survival. Is it possible that the negative effects of profound pain and suffering contribute to the animal's demise? While in veterinary school, the author was exposed to the dogma that "analgesic drugs have dangerous adverse effects and can kill the patient." Although no drug is innocuous, the judicious use of today's available analgesic agents, in accord with accepted professional standards for dosage, route of delivery, and dosing interval for each species, rarely endanger the life of the animal. Although the author is unaware of a scientific study in animals that proves that relief of pain lowers mortality, there are anecdotal reports among veterinarians treating both laboratory and companion animals of improved postprocedural morbidity and mortality with the use of analgesic agents. In a research setting, survivability is increased in animal subjects of burn studies when analgesics are incorporated into the protocol, and companion animals undergoing orthopedic procedures have shown decreased morbidity and mortality when administered postoperative analgesics.

In summary, it is well within the charge of the IACUC to investigate unacceptably high mortality associated with a research study. Many factors can influence experimental mortality, and the committee should dialog with the PI to refine protocols to decrease death in study animals. Relief of pain may be another factor that warrants IACUC attention to determine its influence on improving survivability.

9.13 WHEN SHOULD THE IACUC OBSERVE EXPERIMENTS IN PROGRESS AND/OR REQUEST PILOT STUDIES TO ASSESS PAIN/DISTRESS IN LABORATORY ANIMALS?

Several useful formats are available to resolve the problems that arise when the PI and the IACUC differ on to whether or not a protocol contains painful/stressful methodologies that may require modification. The first suggestion is for a subcommittee of the IACUC to visit the PI's laboratory and observe the experimental manipulations in progress. The subcommittee can be composed of just the attending veterinarian; however, additional members, such as the chairperson and community representative, can be involved. In the opinion of the author, this format presents a nonthreatening and collegial forum for the PI and his or her respective staff to educate the subcommittee members and to prove their case that the procedures are not stressful or noxious to the animals, and thus no protocol modifications are necessary. From the committee's standpoint, their presence in the PI's laboratory sends the message to "show us that the animals will not be in discernable distress and agony and we will get off your back." On the other hand, if the trial before the subcommittee does not go well and the animals are seen to be in obvious distress and discomfort, the IACUC now has objective evidence and is motivated to pursue additional dialog with the PI. The ensuing discussions usually seek protocol modification and elimination of the objectionable methods but may be complicated by the absence of alternatives methodologies that, although more humane, are not optimal to achieve the scientific goals of the project. An example of the latter dilemna involves the continued search for more humane alternatives to Freund's complete adjuvant (FCA) in immunology studies. Although alternative adjuvants often do not produce the localized inflammatory reactions, including abscessation, that are a frequent consequence to the use of FCA, these alternatives may not be as ideal as the FCA in that they may produce a lower humoral antibody titer or even no discernable titer at all, and thus are not scientifically acceptable to fulfill the goals of the project.

Another mechanism available to the committee for resolving protocol issues of possible pain and distress to research animals is to suggest a trial in a small number of animals, often referred to as a pilot study. In this format, the PI is approved, and often encouraged, to conduct the disputed experimental methods in, for example, 25 or less rodents with intensive intra- and postprocedural monitoring for pain and distress by the research, veterinary, and animal-care staffs. Before the pilot study is initiated, objective criteria should be agreed upon by all involved that will be used to assess the animals for loss of condition, pain, and distress throughout the study. Several key criteria, such as distressful vocalization, autotomy (i.e., self-trauma, usually to a limb, that may progress to self-consumption of the extremity), severe aggression in normally placid animals, or a decline in condition to produce a moribund state should also be *proactively* agreed upon before the pilot study begins. When any or all of these conditions are present, the pilot study will be immediately terminated. Other less acute criteria (such as body weight loss, inappetance, resistance to movement) can and should also be agreed upon proactively. As discussed earlier in the chapter, these criteria can often be combined into a pain scoring system (Morton and Griffith, 1984) that will be used in composite to identify whether or not the animals are in pain. The PI should be obliged to promptly report their findings (in writing) to the IACUC before animals can be purchased for the definitive study. This information can then be used as a basis for further constructive dialog between the PI and IACUC, and often provides leverage for both sides to compromise.

In the event that all parties agree that the animals are in distress or suffering, the next step is decide what methods will be agreed upon to reduce their discomfort. This may mean altered experimental methods (such as changes in the animal species, alternative anesthetic methods, or even a change in study design, incorporation of postoperative care measures, analgesic therapy, and an assignment of experimental endpoints including euthanasia). In this manner, a harmonious conclusion to the review process may be reached that permits maximum scientific gain from the study with a smaller degree of discomfort to the experimental animals.

9.14 EXPERIMENTAL ENDPOINTS—SHOULD/MUST DEATH BE AN ENDPOINT OF A RESEARCH STUDY?

All research studies eventually come to some form of conclusion, be it survival and donation of the animal to another approved research project, spontaneous death, or euthanasia. In the past, many research studies concluded with the spontaneous death of the animal, and it was considered crucial for the model that the interval between initiation of the experiment and spontaneous death be calculated. Based on this data, survival curves were generated and were often used to compare therapeutic efficacy of candidate pharmaceuticals. Studies of this nature were particularly challenging and often dreaded by both the research, technical, and animal-care staffs because they involved daily observation of the weakening and debilitation of the study animals until their death.

This format is still in effect for certain scientific specialties but is increasingly being replaced by a format in which the animals are euthanized when a predetermined set of criteria (endpoints) are reached that have shown a strong correlation with impending death. *Particularly in the case of potentially painful procedures performed on laboratory animals, it is important for both the committee and the PI to realize that a time may come in the study when valid scientific data can no longer be gathered owing to the degree of debilitation and alteration from normal physiologic parameters that is present in the animal(s).* In this instance, it is appropriate from both a humane and scientific rationale to terminate the trial. Suggested criteria for signalment that euthanasia is warranted include inappetance such that body weight loss occurs (benchmark is frequently 20 percent body weight loss over the duration of the study), dehydration, debilitation such that movement to reach food and water is impaired, vocalization indicative of severe pain and distress, open, bleeding or infected wounds, tumor growth in excess of 5 percent of the animal's body weight, and dehissance of internal organs (UKCCCR, 1998; Redgate et al., 1991; Olfert, 1995; FELASA Report, 1992; Montgomery, 1990). In addition, some research manipulations provide data (such as hypothermia, profound anemia, and respiratory or cardiovascular collapse) that can, in itself, be predictive of impending death. *In the opinion of the author, it is time well-spent by the committee to negotiate all the fine details of these experimental endpoints during the process of protocol review rather than wait until acute and often emotional circumstances have arisen and try to reach a consensus with the PI at this time.*

9.15   SKILLED/UNSKILLED EUTHANASIA AND ITS RELATIONSHIP TO PAIN AND DISTRESS

Euthanasia literally means "good death . . . that occurs without pain and distress" (AVMA Panel on Euthanasia, 1993). When performed by skilled personnel, euthanasia is a compassionate means to end the life of an animal that is experiencing unmitigated pain and distress during a biomedical research study. In contrast, efforts to perform euthanasia by unqualified personnel or using inappropriate methods or equipment can, in itself, inflict severe discomfort and distress upon an animal. It is the responsibility of the IACUC to assure that all personnel participating in the euthanasia of laboratory animals are competent, use approved methods, and have all required drugs and equipment needed at their immediate disposal to assure that animals truly receive a painless and rapid death. See Appendix J.

9.16   EUTHANASIA GUIDES

IACUCs should educate scientists on recent advances in euthanasia practice or increased knowledge of the consequences of commonly used euthanasia techniques. For example, a recent study suggests that high (70 percent or greater) concentrations of CO_2 gas, when used for euthanasia, may lead to adverse reactions and accompanying pain and distress in rats (Danneman et al., 1997). When indicated, the IACUC may suggest that newly proposed as well as ongoing studies be modified to incorporate recently developed or more humanely acceptable euthanasia methods.

9.17   COMMUNICATION OF THE IACUCS DECISION TO THE PI

Once the protocol has been reviewed and the committee has identified legitimate areas of concern for painful methods therein, the next logical step is to communicate these concerns to the PI and work toward a win–win resolution that benefits both the scientific pursuit and the comfort of the animals. Sometimes, the scientist is unaware that alternative, less painful or distressful methods exist and are accepted in their field (as can be documented by inclusion of these more humane methods in peer reviewed journals and presentation at scientific meetings). When informed that these alternative methods exist, the scientist is happy to accept the requested protocol revisions, the study proceeds uneventfully, and the IACUC has honored its legal and ethical responsibilities to serve as institutional stewards for responsible animal care. The next section of the chapter discusses events that transpire when harmony cannot be easily reached between the PI and the IACUC regarding refinement of methodologies deemed painful.

9.18   COMMUNICATION BARRIERS—WHY ARE SCIENTISTS RESISTANT TO ADDRESSING PAIN MANAGEMENT?

The vast majority of research scientists are highly motivated professionals who abhor the thought of causing unnecessary pain and suffering to an animal. Why then are IACUCs at times faced with resistance from scientists to any form of pain management or protocol modification to refine and, if possible, eliminate painful or stressful methods? Perhaps it is an inherent resistance to change. This may be owing to personal resistance to mess with success or may be owing to fear that they will lose stature and funding by rebelling against time-honored dogmas within their specialty fields. Societal awareness and scrutiny of the use of animals for research purposes has greatly increased over the past decade. The 1985 amendments to the Federal Animal Welfare Act (CFR, Subchapter A, 1985) and the 1986 publication of the PHS policy (Public Health Service, 1986) brought an obligation, often publicly noted, for institutions to commit to animal welfare. For the first time, a peer review process for humane methods (i.e., an IACUC for each licensed institution) was mandated, and research protocols were required before vertebrate animals could be used for studies. Since that time, the *Guide for the Care and Use of Laboratory Animals* (Institute of Laboratory Animal Resources, 1996) was published and has been revised several times. All of these laws and guidelines have promoted change and at times served as educational tools for both the laboratory animal and scientific communities. Scientists lost the freedom to have total control of their research animal use, and past methods have now come under, if not opposition, at least scrutiny for their ability to cause unnecessary pain and suffering to research animals. Some scientific specialties have long held doctrines that death was a required endpoint for their studies and/or that analgesic drug use would unacceptably alter the validity of their studies. In some endeavors, dialog between those supporting animal welfare and the scientific community has brought about refined methodologies and thus harmony between science and humane animal care and use. In others, the road to progress in this area has been less well-traveled.

Where does the responsibility of an IACUC begin and end in asking scientists to consider changing to less distressful experimental methods? First, the committee must understand that the scientists' concerns are at times well-founded. For those investigators dependent upon public funding, it is feasible that study sections and review panels will not favorably review a proposal using newer (although arguably more humane) methods. We are asking quite a lot when pressuring a scientist to abandon the use of time-honored animal models that have repeatedly been a component of federally-funded research projects. What is the cost to science, the advancement of knowledge, and society when leaders in a field are asked to revalidate basic methods and, in the most extreme cases, to essentially begin anew all in the name of animal welfare?

Another common reason that PIs are reluctant to modify a protocol is their belief that the animals are not in pain or distress using the proposed methods. As we all know, animals cannot verbalize their perception of pain and suffering, and for this reason, there can also be contention as to whether or not the animal(s) are actually in pain and truly need any study refinement or analgesic therapy. In some cases, the scientific, veterinary, and animal-care staff are challenged to clearly and unequivocally identify an animal that is, indeed, in pain and, therefore, suffering. It is difficult for an IACUC to require changes in methods that have served a scientist well for many years without objective evidence that the methods cause animal suffering. There are several options for resolving this dilemma short of outright confrontation (which benefits no one, including the animals) between the IACUC and the scientific staff. One of the author's favorite methods is to permit the PI to conduct a small pilot study. A sample format for pilot studies to assess whether or not distress or pain is inflicted in animals used in a research study has been presented earlier in this chapter.

In the rare instance that the PI is resistant to a dialog with the IACUC on any aspect of protocol refinement of clearly inhumane methodologies, the committee and institution should have a formal mechanism in place to disapprove the study until a compromise acceptable to all parties is in place. This is a highly regrettable situation but proceeding with a study of this nature will risk the reputation of the institution and the scientist, and clearly opposes the federal legislation and policies governing animal care and use. Furthermore, studies by Liebeskind and co-workers (Liebeskind, 1991) have shown that unmitigated pain is a bona fide significant scientific variable in its own right (by causing depression of the immune response); thus, it may be of limited scientific value to proceed with the study under these conditions. This is truly a no-win situation for all concerned.

The third major reason, in the opinion of the author, that investigators are reluctant to modify protocols to minimize pain and distress are the logistical problems associated with analgesic drug use. In addition to the concerns discussed previously that the analgesic(s) may compromise the scientific validity of the study, potent pain relieving drugs, such as the opioid analgesics, may be expensive, require a DEA license for purchase, and must be administered multiple times daily often for an indefinite time period. In addition, these drugs are not innocuous and their use may be accompanied by adverse effects. While these are not acceptable justifications for allowing an animal to suffer needlessly when efficacious drugs are available, the IACUC members should recognize that these practical barriers to analgesic drug use do exist. In the opinion of the author, the IACUCs responsibilities do not end with a decree that analgesic drug therapy is needed. Committee members (especially the attending veterinarian who is required by the AWA to consult in protocols that will involve a potential for pain) should be available to work with the PI to offer suggestions for the selection of drug(s), delivery methods, frequency of administration, and management of any untoward adverse effects as well as acceptable methods for drug storage and recordkeeping of controlled substance use. In this manner, a best-fit scenario will be established, benefiting both the animals and the limited resources of the research staff.

9.19 IACUC PROCEDURES TO DISAPPROVE STUDIES AND INVESTIGATE ANIMAL WELFARE COMPLAINTS

The IACUC may be presented with a research protocol that either cannot be modified to minimize severe pain and/or distress or a PI who is unwilling or unable to modify the proposed study to satisfy the committee's humane concerns. In this situation, a mechanism should exist for the committee to disapprove the study—not permit it to commence until a suitable compromise can be worked out.

At other times, there are concerns from employees of the institution that animals were in unrelieved pain and/or distress during a study and sufficient measures were not taken by the responsible individuals to acknowledge and terminate their discomfort. When the latter situation arises, the IACUC should have a mechanism in place for these concerns to be brought before the committee and formats should be available to investigate and subsequently resolve the complaint. (See Chapter 6, Running an IACUC: One Chair's Perspective.) The Federal Animal Welfare Act (CFR, Title 9, Subchapter A, 1985) charges the IACUC with investigating concerns involving the welfare of laboratory animals. Allegations of pain and suffering certainly fall into this category. Reconciling such contentious issues are among the most challenging but most meaningful and productive deliberations that an IACUC will undertake. A format is needed for all parties to provide information in a factual and nonthreatening manner and must include input from the employee that has brought forth the allegation as well as the PI and their respective research staffs. The incident may be investigated by either the full IACUC or a subcommittee, who will in turn report back to the full committee and, if warranted, make recommendations for corrective action. It is the responsibility of the committee to then inform the institutional official and funding agencies if the incident is deemed to be a serious issue of noncompliance and/or the project is suspended. One should remember that the institution's reputation, as well as that of all parties involved, may be at stake, and that any actions taken by the committee should be made in an impartial manner and based solely on protecting the interests of the institution.

9.20   CONCLUSION

In some ways, the measure of an IACUCs worth is its handling of issues of potential pain and distress in research animals. There is no accrediting body guidebook or legislative policy manual that tells the IACUC how to manage a research protocol such that the animals will never hurt or suffer during a study. Furthermore, the animals themselves cannot tell the committee how well it has done its job to keep them comfortable. This chapter has presented what are, in the opinion of the author, the paramount issues to address in protocol review and strategies to resolve issues of potential pain and distress that are mutually beneficial to the animals, scientist, and institution. When these strategies fail, it is appropriate and necessary for the IACUC to investigate and resolve any instances of unnecessary pain and distress in its research animal colony. Rational, open and fair-minded communication between the scientific and animal-care staffs, the IACUC, and those charged with stewardship of institutional compliance are the keystones to the humane care and use of research animals at the institution. Finally, IACUC members should stay current with technological advances and improved methods for the care and treatment of laboratory animals that will facilitate their use in research studies in the most humanely acceptable and scientifically valid manner. When this happens, we are all winners.

REFERENCES

AVMA Panel on Euthanasia, Report of the AVMA panel on euthanasia, *J. Am. Vet. Med. Assoc.,* 202, 230, 1993.

CFR (Code of Federal Regulations), Title 9 (Animals and Animal Products), Subchapter A (Animal Welfare), Office of the Federal Register, Washington, D.C., 1985.

Cornetta, K., Safety aspects of gene therapy, *Br. J. Hema.,* 80, 421, 1992.

Danneman, P. J., Neuroanatomy and neurophysiology of pain, in *Anesthesia and Analgesia in Laboratory Animals,* Kohn, D. F., Wixson, S. K., Benson, J. G., and White, W. J., Eds., Academic Press, New York, 1997, 84, 91.

Danneman, P. J., Stein, S., and Walshaw, S .O., Humane and practical implications of using carbon dioxide mixed with oxygen for anesthesia in euthanasia of rats, *Lab. Anim. Sci.,* 47(4), 376, 1997.

Federation of European Laboratory Animal Science Associations (FELASA) Working Group on Pain and Distress, Pain and distress in laboratory rodents and lagomorphs, *Lab. Anim.,* 28, 97, 1994.

Feldman, S. H. and Hoyt, R. F., A structure for ensuring the safety of gene therapy protocols, *Lab Animal,* 23(5), 44, 1994.

Flecknell, P., *Laboratory Animal Anesthesia,* Academic Press, London, 1996.

Heavner, J. E., Pharmacology of analgesics, in *Anesthesia and Analgesia in Laboratory Animals,* Kohn, D. F., Wixson, S. K., Benson, J. G., and White, W. J., Eds., Academic Press, New York, 1987, 43.

Hubbs, A. F., Designer mice: transgenic and knockout mice in toxicology research, *Lab Animal,* 26, 34, 1997.

Institute of Laboratory Animal Resources, *Guide for the Care and Use of Laboratory Animals,* ILAR Committee, National Research Council, National Academy Press, Washington, D.C., 60, 1996.

Kohn, D. F., Wixson, S. K., Benson, J. G., and White, W. J., Eds., *Anesthesia and Analgesia in Laboratory Animals,* Academic Press, New York, 1997.

Lawrence, M., The unconscious experience, *Am. J. Cri. Care,* 4(3), 227, 1995.

Liebeskind, J. C., Pain can kill, *Pain,* 44, 3, 1991.

Mogil, J. S., Flodman, P., Spence, M. A., Sternberg, W. F., Kest, B., Sadowski, B., Liebeskind, J. C., and Belknap, J. K., Oligogenic determination of morphine analgesic magnitude: a genetic analysis of selectively bred mouse lines, *Behav. Genet.,* 25(4), 397, 1995.

Mogil, J. S., Sternberg, W. F., Marek, P., Sadowski, B., and Belknap, J. K., The genetics of pain and pain inhibition, *Proc. Natl. Acad. Sci. USA,* 93, 3048, 1996.

Montgomery, C. A., Oncologic and toxicologic research: alleviation and control of pain and distress in laboratory animals, *Canc. Bull.,* 42(4), 230, 1990.

Morton, P. B. and Griffith, P. H. M., Guidelines on the recognition of pain, distress and discomfort in experimental animals and an hypothesis for assessment, *Vet. Rec.,* 166, 431, 1984.

National Research Council, The basis of pain, in *Recognition and Alleviation of Pain and Distress in Laboratory Animals,* National Academy Press, Washington, D.C., 1992, 10.

Olfert, E. D., Defining an acceptable endpoint in invasive experiments, *AWIC News.,* 6(1), 3, 1995.

Public Health Service (PHS), Public Health Service Policy on Humane Care and Use of Laboratory Animals, U.S. Department of Health and Human Services, Health Research Extension Act, P.L. 99-158, Washington, D.C., 1986.

Redgate, E. S., Deutsch, M., and Boggs, S. S., Time of death of CNS tumor-bearing rats can be reliably predicted by body weight-loss patterns, *Lab. Anim. Sci.,* 41(3), 269, 1991.

Schnaper, N., The psychological implications of severe trauma: emotional sequelae to unconsciousness, *J. Trauma,* 16(2), 95, 1975.

United Kingdom Co-Ordinating Committee on Cancer Research (UKCCCR), Guidelines for the welfare of animals in experimental neoplasia (2nd ed.), *Br. J. Cancer,* 77(1), 1, 1998.

United States Department of Agriculture (USDA), Annual Report of Research Facility, Animal and Plant Health Inspection Service (APHIS), Form 7023, 1991.

Zimmerman, M., Ethical guidelines for investigations of experimental pain in conscious animals, *Pain,* 16, 109, 1983.

10 IACUC—From a Principal Investigator's Perspective

Robert J. Tressler, Ph.D. and Paula Belloni, Ph.D.

CONTENTS

When Principal Investigators (PIs) first see the forms that have to be filled out for IACUCs, their responses are, "Great! More bureaucratic paperwork to slow me down." But once they gain a better appreciation of the IACUC, the paperwork seems less daunting and they find themselves saying, "It's not that bad."

PIs, sooner or later, come to understand that one of the key roles of an IACUC is to make sure that all studies are carried out in compliance with the Animal Welfare Act. By insisting upon the appropriate care and use of animals, IACUCs effectively keep PIs and the institutions they work for out of trouble. (Infractions of the law could result in the institution and/or investigator being prohibited from carrying out further animal studies that are critical to a research or development program.)

10.1 FILLING OUT THE IACUC PROTOCOL FORM

Before starting studies with animals, PIs must exhaust all possible ways to test an agent in nonanimal systems. If the compound is active, it will have to be tested in an animal model for efficacy and safety before use in humans. At this point, before onset

135

of any studies, the PI must identify the appropriate model system and submit an Animal Care and Use Protocol to the IACUC for review and approval.

The purpose of an IACUC protocol, and having it reviewed by the IACUC, is to make sure that animals will be used in a humane manner that meets the requirements of the Animal Welfare Act. It also helps the PI to focus on the rationale and validity of the proposed study, thereby avoiding any unnecessary and inappropriate use of animals. A properly reviewed and approved protocol shows that the proposal has merit and meets all the specifications of the law; it also "covers" the PI and the institution.

10.2   RESOURCES TO ASSIST THE PI

A variety of internal and external resources are in place to help the PI to fill out IACUC forms. Internal resources include the IACUC itself. Individuals that make up the committee have extensive knowledge about animal protocols and procedures and can help the PI fill out the IACUC form. They can also supply useful scientific input on specific types of models. The IACUC at Roche Bioscience, where one of us works (PB), has a Hint Sheet to guide the PI in filling out forms. Personnel in the vivarium [if the organization has a vivarium in-house] can also assist in drafting specific procedural sections of the IACUC protocol. Another great source for help are other PIs who may already have performed similar studies; they are often willing to supply a copy of their protocols as a reference template.

Valuable external sources are:

1. The *Guide for the Care and Use of Laboratory Animals.*
2. Publications in journals that cite specific model systems related to the area of study.
3. Veterinarians.
4. Databases and information services.

If the PI has drafted a good research plan for the study, with minimal modification much of the research plan can be transferred onto the IACUC form.

10.3   POTENTIAL PITFALLS FOR THE PI

There are specific points in the animal care and use protocol that the PI must adequately describe so that all members of the committee have a good understanding of the nature and appropriateness of the proposed study.

When filling out the protocol, try to write a balanced proposal. You should write the proposal broadly enough to allow for minor alterations in manipulations or treatment. Because the protocol cannot be altered without prior review and approval by the IACUC, try to write in a reasonable amount of latitude about what you intend to do or think you might do in the future. However, you can not be overly generic in your description of animal use. The IACUC must be able to read your protocol and have a complete understanding of the scope of the minor variations that may be incorporated into the proposed series of studies. As a PI on numerous protocols, we have been confronted by IACUCs who felt that our protocol was too vague and too broad. Studies may be delayed when the IACUC asks for more details. In situations where there is some doubt that a procedure will ever be used, it is wiser to omit it, then, later, amend the protocol when something is needed. On the other hand, protocols that are too specific lock in the PI; this may require multiple amendments as changes are needed and can delay studies.

10.4 SELECTED SECTIONS IN THE IACUC PROTOCOL FROM THE PI'S PERSPECTIVE

10.4.1 RATIONALE AND PURPOSE

This section is your chance to tell the committee that your proposal has scientific merit and why it must be carried out in an animal model. Be succinct. Clearly state your overall objectives and how these need to be accomplished using animals. This section primes the IACUC for the review of the rest of your protocol—first impressions are important.

10.4.2 ALTERNATIVES

Obviously, the PI should have exhausted all possible alternatives prior to deciding to perform studies in animals. This is usually achieved by carrying out a literature/scientific survey of alternative models. (See Chapter 11, Literature Search for Alternatives). Such a survey may reward the PI in two ways: first, by providing an alternative method that precludes the need for animal and, second, by identifying the best and most relevant model(s) that may be available.

10.4.3 TRAINING/EXPERIENCE

Another factor the investigator should remember is that the personnel involved in the study must have appropriate training and experience. Documentation of this in the form of training records or a work/experience history of the individuals should be sufficient to assure the committee of this, and can be attached to the protocol. Failing to do this can result in delay of protocol approval. Specific experience on the part of the author has shown this to be the case, with the committee veterinarian often being the person that raises this issue during review of the protocol.

10.4.4 ANIMAL MONITORING—POTENTIAL FOR PAIN AND/OR DISTRESS

This section of the protocol always gets close scrutiny by the committee. It is not uncommon for an investigator to fail to fully address this section if the study that is planned is thought to be an innocuous one with little expectation of distress to the animals. Nonetheless, if there is a chance of any pain or distress to the animals, the investigator must explain how this will be reduced as well as what type and frequency of monitoring will be performed.

10.5   CONCLUSION

The IACUC assists the institution and the PI by supplying expertise in animal care and use and by making sure that the requirements of the Animal Welfare Act and other regulations for animal use are satisfied. The PI should view the IACUC as a resource that can be of great assistance not only from a regulatory standpoint, but also from a scientific and practical standpoint in terms of humane and efficient performance of animal studies.

11 The Literature Search for Alternatives

Michael D. Kreger, M.S.

CONTENTS

". . . the farm bill contains legislation dealing with the humane treatment of animals. The main thrust of the bill is to minimize pain and distress suffered by animals used for experiments and tests. In so doing, biomedical research will gain in accuracy and humanity. We owe much to laboratory animals and that debt can best be repaid by good treatment and keeping painful experiments to a minimum." . . . Senator R. Dole describing what would become the 1985 amendments to the Animal Welfare Act, *Congressional Record*—House, December 17, 1985.

The Improved Standards for Laboratory Animals Act, better known as the 1985 amendments to the Animal Welfare Act, charged each American institution above high school level that conducts biomedical research, teaching, or testing on animals with forming an oversight committee, the Institutional Animal Care and Use Committee (IACUC). Today, among its roles, the IACUC must ensure that principal investigators (PI) have determined that proposed animal studies are not unnecessarily duplicative and that they have considered alternatives to procedures that are likely to cause pain or distress to the animal. PIs must convince the IACUC in writing, usually on the protocol review form, that there are no satisfactory alternatives to the painful procedures proposed and that they have selected the least painful or least stressful procedure that is adequate. While the PI may be an expert in a particular area of research, few are familiar with all of the techniques that can be used to accomplish a research objective. It is therefore not unusual for the IACUC to require an "alternatives search" on the protocol form or to send the protocol back for revision.

Although literature searches have been used to address the alternatives question since 1985, people still ask IACUCs and the U.S. Department of Agriculture's Animal Welfare Information Center, "What is the literature search for alternatives and why do I have to do it?" This is because there are always new researchers entering the field and IACUC memberships change from time to time; some find the idea of the literature search confusing or are unclear about what is required by law and what the benefits may be.

Clarification is available from the USDA office that interprets and enforces the Act, the APHIS/AC. It has issued Animal Care Policies (USDA, May 1997). Policy No. 12 addresses the literature search by clarifying what is meant in the Animal Welfare Act by "written narrative for alternatives to painful procedures." While there are many complicated ways to design and execute a search, this chapter will provide a good starting point for the novice searcher and tips for the researcher and information specialist.

In this chapter we will outline the legislative background and describe how the search for alternatives can best be performed.

11.1   DEFINING ALTERNATIVES

The concept of alternatives was conceived as the three R's by W. M. S. Russell and R. L. Burch (see Reference 6) in their book, *The Principles of Humane Experimental Technique.* The three R's are *R*eduction in number of animals used, *R*efinement of methods to minimize pain and distress to the animals, and *R*eplacement of the animal model with a nonanimal model or a species phylogenetically lower. In doing the literature search, it is important to recognize that alternatives are not just replacing the animal with a computer simulation or an *in vitro* procedure. For example, an improved method of restraining the animal that involves positive reinforcement and minimizes the distress involved in capture and restraint is a refinement alternative. A thorough literature search of articles similar to the proposed study may help determine appropriate animal numbers (e.g., reduction alternative).

11.2   LEGISLATION

The Animal Welfare Act emphasizes minimizing pain and distress. It states in Section 13(a)(3)(B) "that the principal investigator consider alternatives to any procedure likely to produce pain or distress in an experimental animal." Section 13(a)(3)(E) adds a statement about written justification for not adopting an available alternative "that exceptions to such standards may be made only when specified by research protocol and that any such exception shall be detailed and explained in a report outlined under paragraph (7) and filed with the Institutional Animal Committee."

Title 9 of the Code of Federal Regulations presents the USDA regulation on how consideration of alternatives should be accomplished. It includes the Animal Welfare Information Center (AWIC), which relies on multiple database literature searching, as a resource. "[The] IACUC shall determine that . . . the principal investigator has considered alternatives to procedures that may cause more than momentary or slight pain or distress to the animals, and has provided a written narrative description of the methods and sources, e.g., the Animal Welfare Information Center, used to determine that alternatives were not available; . . . ."

The *Federal Register*[1] gives the USDA rationale for making the alternatives consideration a written requirement and suggests a series of databases that can be searched to document whether or not alternatives are available, "The principal investigator must provide a written narrative of the sources, such as Biological Abstracts, Index Medicus, the Current Research Information Service (CRIS), and the Animal Welfare Information Center that is operated by the National Agricultural Library (NAL). We believe that in fulfilling this requirement Committee members will discuss these efforts with the principal investigator in reviewing the proposed activity. We also believe that considerations of alternatives will be discussed during Committee meetings where proposed activities are presented for approval, and made part of the meeting minutes. . . ."

The legislation mandates that the investigator must provide a written narrative that demonstrates to the IACUC that alternatives, useful or not, were at least considered in the experimental design. The literature search is suggested as the best way to demonstrate this. IACUC members, including the nonaffiliated member, a visiting AC inspector, or a member of the public, can follow a printed search strategy, view the list of databases and keywords, and verify that the investigator has made a good faith effort to demonstrate whether or not alternatives exist and why he or she will or will not adopt them. Thus, the literature search is a much better way to judge if alternatives are available than a check-off box or a sentence or two saying there are no alternatives written on the protocol form.

USDA Animal and Plant Health Inspection Service (APHIS)/Animal Care (AC) Policy No. 12, posted on the animal care website (www.aphis.usda.gov/ac/polman.html), was published to help researchers, IACUC members, and other institutional officials understand what the minimum requirements are for consideration of alternatives, as it relates to an electronic database search. It paraphrases the legal statements from 9 CFR and goes on to say, "The minimal written narrative should include: the databases searched or other sources consulted, the date of the search and the years covered by the search, and the key words and/or search strategy used by the Principal Investigator when considering alternatives or descriptions of other methods and sources used to determine that no alternatives were available to the painful or distressful procedure. The narrative should be such that the IACUC can readily assess whether the search topics were appropriate and whether the search was sufficiently thorough. Reduction, replacement, and refinement (the three R's) must be addressed, not just animal replacement."

11.3   SEARCH BENEFITS

Besides the legal mandate in the Animal Welfare Act, there are many other benefits of the alternatives search. The Public Health Service, the U.S. Government *Principles for the Utilization and Care of Vertebrate Animals Used in Testing, Research, and Training;* the Public Health Service policy on *Humane Care and Use of Laboratory Animals* (National Institutes of Health, 1996); and the *Guide for the Care and Use of Laboratory Animals* (National Research Council, 1996) require consideration of alternatives when awarding project funding. Such laws and policies extend to all vertebrates, including those beyond the scope of the Animal Welfare Act. Complying with the Animal Welfare Act and the *Guide for the Care and Use of Laboratory Animals* is required in order for an institution to become accredited by the Association for Assessment and Accreditation of Laboratory Animal Care International (AAALAC).

11.4   HOW TO DO A SEARCH FOR ALTERNATIVES

Strategies for developing and executing the literature search for alternatives have been described by Huggins, 1997; Smith, 1994; Snow, 1990; and Stokes and Jensen, 1995. (See References 3, 7, 8, and 9.) The entire process, however, can be thought of as an inverted pyramid (Figure 11.1). The alternatives search pyramid is a five-step process beginning with the description of the protocol and ending with the written narrative or modification of the proposal. It is inverted because the search incorporates subject fields and techniques with a greater range than the specifics of the protocol might indicate.

The search begins with the researcher describing the protocol. As the search strategy is designed in the second step, the field widens to cover not just the specifics of the protocol, but also methods that can reduce, refine, or replace animal use. The third step is database selection, which involves choosing databases relevant to the researcher's area of interest as well as other databases that may appear tangential. For example, databases might include, in addition to medical databases, a computer technology database that gives computer simulations of a particular procedure. The search is run and evaluated in the fourth step that involves retrieving and evaluating relevant articles. Finally, the search is documented and a written narrative is prepared which describes whether any identified alternatives can or cannot be used. This is probably the broadest step of all in that it should cover all of the three R's. If there is a better way of handling the animal in order to minimize distress, if environmental enrichment can be provided (e.g., group housing for some species), or if an analgesic can provide postoperative comfort to the animal, these should also be reported.

The following example shows how the alternatives search pyramid actually works. Dr. Loewenstein wants to produce polyclonal antibodies in rabbits. He plans to use Freund's complete adjuvant (FCA), which is frequently used to stimulate production of high levels of antibodies in laboratory animals used in research and vaccine production. However, it can also cause severe and painful inflammatory reactions in the animal resulting in peritonitis, granulomas, abcesses, and ulcerating tissue necrosis depending on the injection site (Hanley et al., 1997).

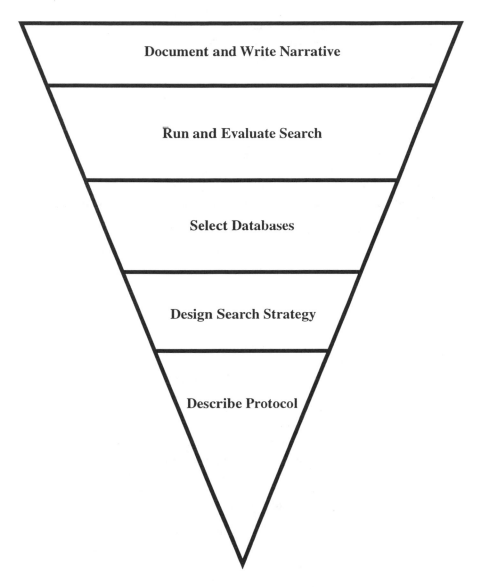

FIGURE 11.1 The Alternative Search Pyramid.

11.4.1 STEP 1: DESCRIBING THE PROTOCOL

Whether Dr. Loewenstein is going to run the search himself or an information specialist or librarian will be running it, describing the protocol is the most important step in developing a search strategy to address alternatives. This is vital to selecting appropriate keywords and databases. Using the antibody example, here are some useful questions to ask the researcher as well as some information that the researcher should convey to the information specialist.

Question: What is the general area of study?
Answer: Polyclonal antibody production.
Question: What species is being proposed?
Answer: Rabbits.
Question: Briefly describe the protocol.
Answer: FCA will be injected intramuscularly into ten rabbits. Dr.
              Loewenstein believes the number of animals and the rabbit model
              will give him the desired level of antibodies. After retrieving the
              antibodies, he will euthanize the animals.
Question: What organ systems or tissues are involved?
Answer: The injection will be intramuscular.
Question: Please name any acronyms and define them as they may be useful
              keywords.
Answer: FCA is used for Freund's complete adjuvant.
Question: Are there any names of hormones, enzymes, generic or trade
              names of compounds, and so on, other than what is already
              described?
Answer: No.
Question: Is this study unique or unnecessarily duplicative?
Answer: While this study is not unique, it is necessarily duplicative because
              further studies will use the antibodies that are produced.
Question: Is the researcher aware of any possible alternatives?
Answer: Dr. Loewenstein suspects there may be *in vitro* techniques and has
              heard of Freund's incomplete adjuvant, but doubts he will get the
              antibody titer level needed.
Question: Were any previous searches run? What databases and keywords
              were used? What were the dates covered?
Answer: Dr. Loewenstein is new to the institution and has not run an alter-
              natives search.

11.4.2   STEP 2: DESIGNING THE SEARCH STRATEGY

There is no one template for designing a search strategy. Smith (1994) uses a two-phase approach, first searching for reduction and refinement techniques, then focusing on replacement in the second phase. Huggins (1997) uses keywords and subject headings provided by database indexers in designing searches. Many librarians use category codes and thesauri provided by individual databases. However, because databases differ by design, the search can be facilitated by searching by keywords only when searching multiple databases. Therefore, in the search design, use words that are likely to appear in the title, abstract, or descriptor fields of the citation. A preliminary search of citations similar to the area of research proposed can also help identify relevant keywords.

The legislation specifically mentions alternatives to the painful procedure; however, the painful procedure must be examined in the context of the entire study. The painful procedures are sometimes, but not often, mentioned in title, abstract, or descriptor categories because the methods information is often buried within the article. Whereas databases do index papers describing methods, most scientists report the results of a study; therefore, alternatives to the painful part of the procedure may require reading sections from articles. A broader view is needed to see if the study's ultimate objectives can be met with alternative methods.

Searching for appropriate animal numbers (reduction) can also be built into the alternatives search. By running an alternatives search, citations are retrieved that cover studies similar to the one proposed. Animal numbers are often found in the materials and methods sections of the articles. The proposed number can also be justified by consulting with a statistician.

In toxicology testing, the search is easily run if the type of compound is known. If the test compound is unknown or if certain tests are required by other federal agencies, it is important to remember that alternatives means more than simply searching for a replacement technique. The investigator can search for a method that uses fewer animals, where mortality is not the endpoint, or search for techniques that minimize pain or distress by using analgesics. Even environmental enrichment can be considered a refinement.

In the case of Dr. Loewenstein's polyclonal antibody production, the search strategy could include keywords such as "polyclonal," "antibody," or "production" in one search statement. The next statement can include the animal model "rabbit" to determine what similar work has been done using this model. If there are ways to minimize pain and distress (refinement) in the rabbit or reduce the number (reduction) of rabbits necessary, "rabbit" is a keyword that must be included. The same line could include words like "alternative," "vitro," "culture," "model," or any other potential alternative that the researcher or information specialist can think of (replacement). Because it is known that polyclonal antibody production is a rapidly growing field, the search could be further limited to contain words like "technique," "method," or "procedure."

If Dr. Loewenstein is using DIALOG, an online database system, Table 11.1 shows how this search strategy might appear.

11.4.3   STEP 3: SELECTING DATABASES

There is no right or wrong number of databases to select when running an alternatives search. The search is a performance, not an engineering, standard. (A performance standard is based on the user deciding how to get to a desired outcome; an engineering standard gives specific requirements for how to get to the same outcome.) As a performance standard, there is no minimum or maximum number of databases required for a search. It is important to recognize that no single database reviews all the literature in all research fields. Databases do overlap somewhat in the journals they index and the subject areas they cover, but they also complement each other. Testing a new medical device, for example, might involve searching biomedical, engineering, and even computer sciences databases. The objectives of the search are to demonstrate whether alternatives are available and, if so, are they useful? A thorough search always requires more than one database.

Bibliographic databases provide the foundation for a good search for alternatives. With the exception of more historic literature (before 1966), they have virtually

---

TABLE 11.1
An Example of a Dialog Search

If Dr. Loewenstein is using DIALOG, an online database system, this is how that search strategy in a multiple database search might appear.

S1   (polyclonal (w) antibod? (4n) produc?)/ti,de
S2   (rabbit? or alternative? or vitro or culture? or model? or simulat? or adjuvant?)/ti,de
S3   S1 and S2
S4   S3 and PY = 1990:1998
S5   S4 and (technique? or method? or procedure?)/ti,de
S6   rd
S7   S6 and (S1 or S2)/ti

Although every online database system has its own syntax for searching, most are very similar. In DIALOG, "w" keeps words in the order written, "4n" keeps words in the order written or reversed, and allows up to 4 words in between. "?" is used as truncation so "simulat?" which will give "simulate," "simulation," etc. "ti,de" keeps the keywords in titles and descriptors, which is very useful if there are many articles on the subject and you are most interested in methods or procedure articles. "PY" indicates a range of publication years. The publication years selected represent when the researcher or information specialist believes new techniques or validated alternatives are most current. To remove duplicate citations in overlapping databases, DIALOG uses the command "rd."

---

replaced printed journal indexes. Usually, bibliographic databases are collections of article citations, with or without abstracts, from hundreds of subject-related journals. It is important to recognize, when selecting databases, what kinds of publications are indexed in each. Some include journal articles only, whereas others also include conference proceedings, audiovisuals, book chapters, and reports. Each citation includes the title, author, year of publication, publisher, and keyword descriptors. These, plus abstracts, are usually prepared by the authors or may be specially written by the database producer.

Bibliographic databases can be searched on compact disk (CD-ROM) or on a multidatabase computer system. Compact disk advantages include: for an annual subscription fee, there is no charge for search time, downloading, or printing records, and the disk can be used on any computer with a CD-ROM drive. Disadvantages include: only one database can be searched at a time; each disk covers a small number of publication years—very much like MEDLINE disks that cover a single publication year; and subscriptions must be maintained to multiple CD titles because no one CD-ROM title adequately covers the entire alternatives literature.

Multidatabase computer systems (online database services) also have their advantages and disadvantages. An annual subscription fee entitles you to access and search several databases simultaneously. A specific publication year or range of years can be searched and duplicate citations can be removed from overlapping databases. Although an online search can be quick and simple, fees are charged for each database accessed, the print format, and downloading (e.g., it is more expensive to download a citation with its abstract than without), the number of citations printed, and the amount of time spent on the online system. Charges can range from tens to hundreds of dollars

TABLE 11.2
Databases for Searching for Alternatives Include the Following with Their Dialog File Numbers

Biomedical and Biological

AGRICOLA	10
AGRIS International	203
ASFA Aquatic Sciences & Fisheries Abstracts	44
BIOSIS Previews 1985+	55
CAB Abstracts	50
EMBASE 1985+	72
Life Sciences Collection	76
MEDLINE 1985+	154
PsychINFO: Psychological Abstracts	11
SciSearch: A Cited Reference Database 1988+	34
TOXLINE	156
Zoological Record Online	185

Federally-Funded Research

CRIS/USDA	60
Federal Research in Progress (FEDRIP)	266
NTIS: National Technical Information Service	6

Pharmaceutical

International Pharmaceutical Abstracts	74
Pharmaceutical News Index	42
Registry of Toxic Effects of Chemical Substances (RTECS)	336

Teaching and Education

A-V Online	46
ERIC	1
MicroComputer Software Guide OnLine	278
Philosopher's Index	57

Technology, Engineering, Medical Devices

Ei Compendex	8
INSPEC 1969+	2
Microcomputer Abstracts	233
NTIS: National Technical Information Service	6

depending on the specificity of the search. The online database service used by the Animal Welfare Information Center and many university and research industry libraries is DIALOG (see Table 11.2). Anyone with an Internet connection can subscribe to the DIALOG service, establish a valid ID and password, and obtain access privileges.

There are hundreds of bibliographic databases, so selecting ones relevant to your search topic is very important. If you know a journal that contains some of the relevant articles, you can begin selecting databases by looking for the list of databases that include the journal's articles. The list is usually found near

Guidelines for Authors or just inside the cover. Another way of finding where a journal is indexed is to do a title search in DIALOG Journal Name Finder, file 414 (DIALOG databases are numbered as files).

For Dr. Loewenstein's polyclonal antibody search, the databases chosen are AGRICOLA, MEDLINE, TOXLINE, EMBASE, and BIOSIS Previews. When duplicate citations are removed, the citations that remain in the list are those that appear first. Therefore, it is more economical to list the less expensive, federally-funded, databases first. Although DIALOG does not charge for viewing titles only, the current (1998) cost for listing a bibliographic citation without the abstract is $0.70 in AGRICOLA, $0.20 in MEDLINE, $0.70 in TOXLINE, $1.45 in BIOSIS Previews, and $1.90 in EMBASE. The costs increase when abstracts are viewed with citations. (Caveat: Prices change from time to time.)

In this search, AGRICOLA was selected because it indexes journals dealing with alternatives, laboratory animal care and use, and veterinary medicine from cover to cover and selectively indexes many other related conference proceedings, reports, audiovisuals, and newsletters. AGRICOLA is produced by the National Agricultural Library (NAL). Because AWIC is located at NAL, AGRICOLA contains much of the recent alternatives literature. AGRICOLA is the only database to index all of AWIC's publications, including its bibliographies and the *Animal Welfare Information Center Bulletin.*

MEDLINE and TOXLINE are produced at the National Library of Medicine (NLM); they overlap in coverage and emphasis. These and other NLM databases (e.g., CANCERLIT and AIDSLINE) cover human and laboratory animal medical journals and selectively index veterinary medical journals. They do not index reports, audiovisuals, or conference proceedings. The alternatives literature found in MEDLINE comes from peer-reviewed medically-related journals. MEDLINE and the other databases produced by NLM are available on CD-ROM, as well as by a direct end-user service called GRATEFUL MED. By using GRATEFUL MED software, a personal computer and a telephone line, individual users can dial up and search the bibliographic database themselves for timely, up-to-date medical information. MEDLINE is also available free of charge on the World Wide Web.

While many researchers search MEDLINE for alternatives, few realize that EMBASE covers the same subject areas with very little citation overlap. It is the experience of AWIC staff members that no alternatives search that uses MEDLINE is complete without also searching EMBASE. EMBASE, produced by Elsevier Science Publishers, includes citations and abstracts from articles and conference proceedings. Over 3500 journals are indexed.

BIOSIS Previews is the electronic version of Biological Abstracts. It indexes over 10,000 books, articles, reports, and conference proceedings. For general natural history information, behavior, and animal welfare studies, BIOSIS is a very comprehensive database and includes many of the citations found in the database Zoological Record. Both databases are also available on CD-ROM.

11.4.3.1 Other Methods and Sources

Whereas online database searching provides the best starting point for searching for alternatives, it must be remembered that there are databases and web sites that cannot be reached via an online database system. There are other sources capable of providing a wealth of alternative-related material that can supplement the literature search. A good example is the web site Altweb, which is produced by the Johns Hopkins Center for Alternatives to Animal Testing (CAAT) as a collaborative project with industry, government, and humane organizations. It contains alternatives news, education resources, and scientific and regulatory information. Conference proceedings (e g , monoclonal antibody production), full text articles, and links to other sites are included.

Norwegian Reference Centre for Laboratory Animal Science and Alternatives produces NORINA, which contains a list with descriptions and ordering information for over 3600 audiovisuals. Audiotapes, CD-ROMs, computer simulations and other programs, films, and models are listed. This searchable web-based database is particularly useful for those seeking alternatives to or supplements for using animals in teaching and training protocols.

Alternatives in Education Database is a downloadable database on the Web produced by the Association of Veterinarians for Animal Rights (AVAR). It contains a list of simulations, models, and aids for primary school to medical and veterinary school courses. Subjects range from alternatives to dissection to microvascular surgery. The database can also be ordered on diskette from AVAR.

PREX is produced at the Department of Laboratory Animal Science, Utrecht University, the Netherlands. It is a subscription-based system that contains major databases like AGRICOLA, CAB, MEDLINE, and Life Sciences as well as very useful additional databases such as AT Alternatives (a German database), Biological Values, Biomedical Dissertations, Book Contents, Current Contents, and more. Also included are VETDOSER, which contains dosages of veterinary medicines, and Strain Sources, which lists strains, descriptions, and sources for inbred mice and rats. Some of these databases are only available through the PREX system.

The PRIMATES database is the most comprehensive information on nonhuman primates and is produced by the Primate Information Center, University of Washington. The Center offers custom searches and also leases PRIMATES with some restrictions on its use. Leasing fees are negotiated by the Center.

STEP 4: EXECUTING AND EVALUATING THE SEARCH

Once the search is executed and downloaded or printed, the PI must review the information and make the determination whether or not alternatives are available. If they are, can they be used? In some instances, the PI might know from the title of the citation whether or not the article is relevant to the particular protocol; however, there will probably be citations that the PI will have to look up in order to read the entire article. This is especially true when animal numbers and methods appear in the materials and methods sections but are not described in the abstract.

In Dr. Loewenstein's search, 266 unique citations were found. Most of the databases searched included some unique citations that appear relevant to alternatives in polyclonal antibody production. No single database provided all of the citations. Samples include:

- From AGRICOLA: reduction in animal numbers required for antisera production using the subcutaneous chamber technique in rabbits.
- From MEDLINE: a comparison of antibody responses to veterinary vaccine antigens potentiated by different adjuvants.
- From EMBASE: evaluation of subcutaneous chambers as an alternative to conventional methods of antibody production in chickens.
- From BIOSIS Previews: production of polyclonal antibodies in rabbits.

Dr. Loewenstein must decide if anything found in the citation list is indeed a viable alternative for his project. He will have to read some of the articles to make that determination. The literature search coupled with findings from other sources used (e.g., web sites, conferences attended, personal training, and experience) will help him reach a decision. He may find useful alternatives such as a way to house the animals that is more comfortable or an analgesic given to relieve pain caused by the adjuvant. There may also be a way to get the desired antibody levels with fewer animals. The bottom line is that the researcher must use the search to convince the IACUC members that the proposed study plan is the most humane way to meet the objectives of the study. If an alternative is found, it should be identified and considered for the protocol.

11.4.5   STEP 5: DOCUMENTING THE ALTERNATIVES
SEARCH AND WRITING THE NARRATIVE

There is no universal standard or template for documenting alternatives searches. Some protocol forms contain a section that asks the researcher to describe efforts to determine if alternatives are available. At a minimum, the researcher must provide the search strategy or keywords used, the databases searched, and the publication years covered. In DIALOG, the command SHOW FILES will list the databases searched with the publication years covered by the databases. Publication years can be further limited in the search strategy as in Dr. Loewenstein's search. The search strategy is displayed by typing DS for DISPLAY SETS.

Some IACUCs ask researchers to attach a copy of the search whereas others suggest the researcher keep it on file for future reference. Any other methods used to supplement the literature search, such as web sites, consultations with experts, or conferences attended, should also be mentioned on the protocol form. If an alternative is found that is useful, but not relevant for this particular project, PIs must justify, in writing, why it cannot be used.

Because the IACUC records of some facilities can be accessed by the public, the literature search can be viewed not only as good science, but also good public relations. The literature search provides a good faith effort on the part of the researcher to demonstrate that the research is as humane as possible and it reflects well on the institution. Alternatives may be found that can lead to adoption of experimental methods that are less painful, use fewer animals, and make better scientific and economic sense. If alternatives are not found, the search demonstrates that there is no other way and no more humane way to do the research than what is proposed.

11.5   TIME AND MONEY

Searches with more specific keywords (e.g., chemical compound names, known alternatives, species being proposed) take less time than very broad generic online searches. Online searching time can be reduced by preplanning the search strategy on paper or using CD-ROMs. Keeping each concept in the search in separate sets or lines helps save money because sets can later be combined. If all concepts are put into a single search set, then any modifications (e.g., removing or adding concepts) require the whole search to be retyped and rerun. With the assistance of a librarian, information specialist, or AWIC staff member, a search strategy can be designed that minimizes time online.

Somebody has to pay the cost for searching. Many university and company libraries give students and staff free access to online databases. MEDLINE is available free of charge on the World Wide Web. Some database systems like PREX offer unlimited use of a set of databases for one subscription fee. Other online systems, like DIALOG, have a yearly fee that gives access to hundreds of databases, but there are additional fees associated with using each database every time you log on. CD-ROMs are another option that involves subscription fees only. A comprehensive DIALOG search run by AWIC costs between $20 to $300 depending on the nature of the protocol. Some facilities have included literature search costs as part of their operating budget or the costs are built into grant or study proposals.

11.6   CONCLUSION

Many researchers run literature searches when designing a study. This helps determine if the research is original or unnecessary duplication (which must be documented) and provides background information on the topic of interest. Such searches can easily be tailored to address alternatives. The search shows that the researcher will stand behind his or her work and that it is as humane as possible. Sometimes, the adoption of an alternative method is more economical, for example, using an *in vitro* model vs. housing a colony of animals. It may provide more meaningful data by avoiding confounding factors in the experimental design, such as distress in the animal model. With a little patience and understanding, researchers will see the alternatives search as a valuable tool for improving the quality of research.

SOURCES AND SUGGESTED READING

1. Animal welfare, final rules, Part IV, *Federal Register,* Vol. 54, No. 168, August 31, 1989.
2. Hanley, W. C., Bennett, B. T., and Artwohl, J. E., Overview of adjuvants, in *Information Resources and Antibody Production,* Smith, C., Jensen, D., Allen, T., Kreger, M., Eds., Beltsville, MD, 1997, 1.
3. Huggins, J., Communication by keyword: sharing information about alternatives to animal testing, *Animal Welfare Information Center Newsletter,* 8(2), 9, 1997.
4. National Academy of Sciences, *Guide for the Care and Use of Laboratory Animals,* National Academy Press, Washington, D.C., 1996.

5. National Research Council, Office of the Director, Public Health Service Policy on Humane Care and Use of Laboratory Animals, Office for Protection from Research Risks, National Institutes of Health, Rockville, MD, 1996.

6. Russell, W. M. S., and Burch, R. L., *The Principles of Humane Experimental Technique,* Universities Federation for Animal Welfare, Herts, England, 1959, reprinted 1992.

7. Smith, C., AWIC tips for searching for alternatives to animal research and testing, *Lab Animal,* 23, 46, 1994.

8. Snow, B., Online searching for alternatives to animal testing, *Online,* July, 94, 1990.

9. Stokes, W. S. and Jensen, D. J. B., Guidelines for Institutional Animal Care and Use Committees: consideration of alternatives, *Contemp. Top.,* 34(3), 51, 1995.

10. Title 7, U.S. Code (1997), Animal Welfare Act as Amended, Sec. 2131 et seq.

11. Title 9, Code of Federal Regulations (1996), Chapter 1, Subchapter A, Animal Welfare.

12. USDA/APHIS/AC, Policy Number 12, Written narrative for alternatives to painful procedures, in *Animal Care Policies,* May 1997. Available from USDA/APHIS/AC, 4700 River Road, Unit 84, Riverdale, MD 20737-4981.

12 Ethics and Quandaries

CONTENTS

Keenly aware that the Constitution would never answer all the questions that might arise in the new United States of America, our founding fathers provided mechanisms to resolve disputes and interpret the laws. Similarly, the AWA tried to cover all contingencies in its rules and regulations but invariably situations have arisen that fall between the cracks. IACUCs must devise suitable ways to handle them. It is incumbent for IACUCs to realize that these problems exist and to resolve them in a manner best suited for their institutions and environments. All authors of this book have contributed some of their perplexing experiences to this chapter.

0-8493-2580-3/99/$0.00+$.50
© 1999 by CRC Press LLC

12.1   EVALUATIONS OF SCIENTIFIC MERIT

The AWA never authorized IACUCs to interfere with the design and scientific method of a study. Nonetheless, the National Institutes of Health as well as the Federation of American Societies for Experimental Biology (FASEB) have asked IACUCs to review the relevance of proposed research. PHS policy states that procedures should be "consistent with sound research design" and "be designed . . . with due consideration of their relevance to human or animal health, the advancement of knowledge, or the good of society."

Does an IACUC have an ethical responsibility to assess the merits of any project that comes before it?

Dr. Wixson believes that this is occasionally warranted—when either intradepartmental "discretionary" funds or "leftover" monies from large extramural sources would fund a study. In this circumstance, the actual research project is not peer reviewed for scientific validity by the NIH or any other extramural expert panel, although, arguably, the scientific merit of the project has been reviewed and funds have been approved by the department head.

See additional comments by Dr. Schiffer in Chapter 4.

12.2   BIOETHICS

How do IACUCs balance the use of animals in research against societal benefits of biomedical research? Do religious beliefs influence how we use animals in research? Do animals have a moral status because they are sentient? What are the ethical issues surrounding genetic engineering research? These issues and others were discussed at the 1998 American College of Laboratory Animal Medicine (ACLAM) forum, "Bioethics and the Use of Laboratory Animals: Ethics in Theory and Practice." A publication summarizing the discussions is available through ACLAM (http://www.aclam.org). It is edited by A. Lanny Kraus, David Renquist, and Jerrold Tannenbaum.

12.3   CONTRACT RESEARCH
ORGANIZATIONS/COLLABORATIONS

Owing to many factors such as downsizing, the high cost of research, increased complexity of research models, and so on, private companies and universities are contracting out more research or forming collaborations with other institutions. Does the IACUC need to be involved and, if so, what are its responsibilities? Ownership of the animals is a critical issue. According to the AAALAC, if the sponsoring institution legally owns the animals, it is responsible and the IACUC must review their use. If the other institution owns the animals, should the sponsoring institution's IACUC still be involved? Does the other institution even have an IACUC? If it is AAALAC accredited, it does. To be cautious, the sponsoring institution's IACUC should be informed of contract and collaborative studies and should at least have some assurance that the other institution has a functional IACUC that will review the use of all animals at their institution. Additional guidelines will be provided in the future by the AAALAC.

12.4   TURF DISPUTES

Veterinarians and investigators often find themselves in conflict with each other. For example, some investigators would prefer to keep small animals in their laboratory for close, frequent observations, but, if these rooms do not conform to the standards for light, temperature, and sanitation found in animal rooms, the veterinarian must disallow this practice. At times, investigators may be reluctant to euthanize an animal at the veterinarian's request because it would disrupt their statistical design. Should the IACUC assume a judicial role?

If the IACUC fails to do this, who will? The veterinarian should not be forced to take a stance that is unsupported by the IACUC (not because the committee disagrees with him/her, but because the committee refuses to address the issue). In this manner, have we not turned the veterinarian into the "lone institutional wolf" crying for animal welfare?

The consensus states that there is a need for a dialog between the PI, the veterinarian, and the IACUC to address and solve issues about euthanasia. It is one of the most important jobs of the committee. If the committee refuses to enter this arena, they have reduced themselves to "paper pushers," not guardians of institutional welfare.

12.5   TRANSFERRING ANIMALS TO A LABORATORY OR OTHER SITE THAT IS NOT APPROVED FOR HOUSING

Although the AWA is pretty specific about keeping animals in locales other than those approved for housing, investigators often present convincing arguments for keeping animals in their laboratories: "We can watch them closer." "We need to work with them every six hours for a week and we need to do the work in our lab because we are not allowed to move our large electronic monitoring equipment into the animal holding room."

Should the IACUC bend the rules even if environmental conditions such as temperature, air exchange, and light cycles are similar to those in the animal facility? Who is responsible for ensuring the animals are monitored daily, provided with fresh food and water, and their cages are properly sanitized? What other activities occur in the laboratory that may affect the animals?

12.6   UNDUE PRESSURES

The protocol of the chief of surgery at a university's medical center has just failed to gain approval by the university's IACUC because the study proposed death as an endpoint. The surgeon brings his grievance to the dean. The dean, aware of the large amount of income that the surgeon generates, advises the IACUC to reconsider its action. If the IACUC reverses its stand, then it is submitting to undue pressure; if it sticks to its guns, then the dean, as the institutional officer, can legally appoint a new committee. Either way, the IACUC loses.

Because IACUCs include members who are researchers at the institution, conflict may arise when a member criticizes a protocol submitted by a superior, commanding officer (in military installations), or a colleague. Often, IACUC members are researchers who are required to serve a period of time on the committee on a rotational basis. The member, aware that the appointment is temporary, may be reluctant to criticize a protocol of a researcher who may be his or her replacement in the future.

For many years, the Lethal Dose 50 (LD_{50}) was the established measure of mean value—that is, the dose of an experimental compound that, when administered to animals, results in 50 percent mortality. Recently, modifications to this concept have been developed and alternatives have become available. Lethal Dose 50 tests are no longer necessary. Some investigators, however, insist that death as an endpoint provides useful information. Who gives in, investigator or IACUC? See Dr. Wixson's Chapter 9, The Role of the IACUC in Assessing and Managing Pain and Distress in Research Animals, for a discussion on death as an endpoint.

12.7   CONFLICT OF INTEREST

This is related to undue pressures. A biologist, Brenda, is the toxicology department's representative on the IACUC. Her boss has a protocol before the IACUC that states that moribund animals will be euthanized. Brenda knows that this investigator does not euthanize animals in a timely manner but prefers to keep them in the study for as long as possible for statistical reasons. If Brenda brings this information to the IACUC and the protocol is shot down, Brenda may face retribution; if she fails to speak out, she is abrogating her IACUC responsibilities. Should such people get the same anonymity and protection that is afforded to other whistle-blowers?

12.8   TOE AND TAIL CLIPPING

Toe clipping is employed as a means of identification. Tail clipping provides tissues for molecular analysis to determine the presence or absence of a particular gene sequence in transgenic rodents.

Justification for toe clipping rests on the premise that pain in the neonate is minimal and momentary—no worse than a needle prick for an injection or blood withdrawal. Furthermore, stringent AWA directives are not applicable to lab rats and mice. (Gerbils, hamsters, etc., are covered by AWA.) (They are, however, applied to all vertebrates through the Public Health Service policy and AAALAC International Standards.) But alternatives such as ear notching, ear tagging, implantable transponders, freeze branding, and tattooing are traumatic, time consuming, and often less effective.

As a means of obtaining tissue for analysis, the questions arise: is it not preferable to obtain tissues by other means, or is it possible to anesthetize the animals for this procedure? Some IACUCs question these practices, especially for identification purposes, in light of recent studies that indicate that pain thresholds increase with neonatal age, and that human neonates, of all gestational ages, do indeed experience nociception and pain response.

Also, should the IACUC concern itself with the feelings of technicians who perform clippings day after day?

12.9 TRANSGENIC AND GENE KNOCKOUT ANIMALS

Genetic manipulation technology is a potent tool for developing animal models of human diseases. Since infectious agents may manifest themselves differently in transgenic animals, a way must be found to closely monitor them for microbial contamination. Additionally, we must be alert to the undue pain and suffering that might result from genetic alterations.

Can IACUCs develop a mechanism for monitoring newly developed strains and guidelines for minimizing or preventing pain and distress?

Other quandaries: everyone agrees that a protocol is needed to create transgenic animals, but is a protocol necessary to breed these transgenics? If toe and tail clipping is required, which protocol should include these procedures? If an investigator breeds his or her transgenic mice and uses them for research and also transfers some of them to other PIs, does the IACUC know which protocols they are used under?

12.10 XENOTRANSPLANTATION

Implanting tissues or whole organs across species introduces the possibility of introducing xenogenic infections that could crossover into man. Should IACUC members take it upon themselves to monitor, even disallow, such infectious Russian roulette? What about the animals that might suffer severe symptoms of rejection? Can painkillers alone alleviate the pain and suffering that accompanies acute and chronic graft rejection?

12.11 DEPARTURES FROM STANDARD OPERATING PROCEDURES

Many institutions have adopted AAALAC's procedural recommendations as their official Laboratory Animal Resource/IACUC guide. If investigators depart from these rules, their protocols will fail to gain approval—despite being in the best interest of the animals. Here is a case in point.

An IACUC's guide states that nonhuman primates shall not be restrained in a chair for more than eight hours. An employee who regularly tests the metabolism of new drugs on nonhuman primates at 8, 10, and 12 h intervals reports that, "At the end of eight hours I can use ketamine to take the test animals out of the chair, put them into cages, and two and four hours later subject them to ketamine again for further sample collection. Wouldn't it be easier to stretch the guidelines, keep the animals in chairs longer, and forgo the need for repeated ketamine administrations?"

How and when to stretch the rules is problematic for all IACUCs. But only by questioning our rules and guidelines can progress be made—perhaps finding a more humane way of doing things.

12.12   ANIMAL ORGAN/TISSUE HARVEST

If an investigator uses live animals to obtain parts or tissues, unquestionably, a protocol and IACUC approval is required. If parts or tissues are obtained from a slaughterhouse, certainly, no protocol is required. However, when parts or tissues are used from animals euthanized for some other purpose, questions arise. Some IACUCs exempt this use from protocol requirements; others insist upon a protocol and review process.

One of the writers of this book responded:

"I have no problem with an investigator inheriting tissues from animals that are euthanized for another purpose; in fact, I encourage it to reduce the number of animals used at my institution. I do not believe a protocol is required if the tissues will truly be inherited from an investigator that would have euthanized the animal(s) for another approved study and purpose. The animal use has already been justified and the animal has already given its life for an approved study—I'm merely authorizing the donation of additional tissues that would have otherwise been discarded."

Presumably, right and wrong hinges upon intent.

12.13   THE LITERATURE SEARCH

The librarian reports that some investigators ask the librarian to do a literature search on specific or alternate procedures, but after the full report has been prepared, it is disregarded, even unread. How can the IACUC be sure that a valid search was done and its information properly weighed—despite the fact the investigator claims to have made a comprehensive search and attaches photocopies of the (librarian's) database reports?

As one author of this book put it, "I really get ticked off when I see canned statements like 'only a living organism' is suitable for this study and computer simulations are not adequate. Animal numbers have been devised to predict statistical significance." Such disclaimers, in today's research environments, imply that the PI put little or no thought or effort into the search (see USDA Policy No. 12 in Chapter 1, and Chapter 11, The Literature Search for Alternatives).

12.14   MEETING CRITERIA OF OTHER AGENCIES

The Food and Drug Administration requires that certain types of studies be performed in at least two mammalian species, of which one is a nonrodent. Additionally, duplication is required to validate screening assays, and no one is certain that *in vitro* screening systems are 100 percent predictive of what will happen in a mammalian system. How can IACUCs reduce animal usage and still comply with requirements of other agencies? Perhaps through refinement techniques we can find a solution.

12.15   ALTERNATIVE THERAPIES

Many veterinarians consider acupuncture to be a viable treatment option in veterinary medicine. Should such alternative therapies be encouraged by the IACUC in studies where analgesics cannot be administered? For instance, experiments designed to evaluate analgesics preclude the administration of painkilling drugs to experimental animals. Should we not try alternative therapies on animals to reduce pain and suffering?

12.16   MULTIPLE SURGERIES

While studying the effects of urethral constrictions in pigs, the principal investigator, during the initial surgery, attaches a urethral ring and implants telemetry devices for the measurement of bladder contractions. But sometimes the constriction becomes totally occlusive and the animal may not survive without surgical intervention. The IACUC permits another surgery to relieve the obstruction, but if the animal survives, should it be subjected to subsequent surgeries to try to salvage the model? Should the animal be euthanized? To put it another way, is it wiser to do multiple surgeries on a few animals or a single surgery on many animals?

Veterinarians are allowed to perform routine veterinary procedures to save animal lives. If the veterinarian relieves the occlusion by performing an emergency surgery, is the veterinarian not in compliance with IACUC policies?

12.17   PILOT STUDIES

Dr. Jones does a complete literature search but can find no model for his contemplated study of bowel distention in pigs. He asks the veterinarian to transfer to him any pigs that are left over from training sessions (covered by training protocols) in order to try a novel, nonrecovery experimental surgery. Since this bypasses the critical purview of IACUC, should it be allowed? And if disallowed, what is to prevent Dr. Jones from "borrowing" a pig from one of his approved protocols for this purpose? How does the IACUC cope with juggling of animals? (See Chapter 9, The Role of the IACUC in Assessing and Managing Pain and Distress in Research Animals.)

12.18   STERILE INJECTIONS

The toxicology staff inject nonsterile experimental compounds (just as they come from the laboratories) into animals. When questioned by the IACUC they respond, "We have never observed any infections."

"If we insist on strict sterility with surgery," says the IACUC, "shouldn't we insist on sterile injections?" "Not so," reply the toxicology people. "Autoclaving or using other sterilizing agents might alter the test substance, thereby invalidating the tests." Who is right?

The response of several authors went something like this:

The issue here is really trying to ensure that the animal responds to the compound being injected and nothing else (such as bacteria, molds, and irritating chemicals in the injectate). We have found many researchers who are willing to filter injectates, which, depending on the size of the millipore, etc., used, will exclude bacteria, fungi, and spores from being introduced into the animal. Viruses are often not excluded by filtering; however, most of the viral pathogens we are concerned with, that will harm animals, are not present in scientific laboratories. We have found this approach to be particularly effective with antibody production in rabbits, which is a process where a variety of substances are mixed with the adjuvant and injection leads to abscessation. The removal of contaminants by filtering often leads to a lesser degree of postinjection sequelae that requires veterinary care and often delays the next booster injection.

12.19   EXPEDITED REVIEW OF A MINOR PROTOCOL AMENDMENT

A principal investigator asks the IACUC chair to use his authority to quickly approve a protocol amendment that presents a minor change. The chair has accommodated PIs in the past when protocols were in the C category, but this happens to be an E protocol, so the chair demurs. The PI then reminds him, "You can do it. There is nothing in the law that requires approval of a minor amendment by the full IACUC." But the chair counters, "the crux of the matter lies in the definition of *minor.* Think of ham and eggs. What is minor for the chicken is hardly so for the pig."

12.20   TEACHING PROTOCOLS

The facility's veterinarian gives several classes on one operative technique and submits the proper teaching protocols. Some IACUC members consider this to be unnecessary duplication. "Hold one class instead of four," they say. The DVM replies, "Only in small hands-on classes do the students benefit from the experience." When are teaching protocols really unnecessarily duplicative?

12.21   DUPLICATIONS

While on the subject of duplicative teaching protocols, the question arises: should the IACUC insist that investigators contact other researchers with a proven scientific model before they try to reproduce results on their own in-house model? This also applies to pilot studies.

12.22   FUNDING AGENCY REQUISITES

A funding agency firmly insists on the use of animals for the studies it supports. A literature search reveals that a new cell culture method that accomplishes everything that the animal models did has recently been published. This is brought to the attention of the funding agency but they will not budge. "Our guidelines were set (several years ago) by expert consultants. Perhaps next year's budget will allow us to reevaluate our guidelines." Do you wait or use the new technique and risk losing all funding?

12.23   EFFECTS ON PERSONNEL

Should the IACUC concern itself with the psychological and occupational effects that experiments are going to have on the people doing the experiment? Indeed, many institutions offer grief counseling for animal care and research personnel. (See Section 12.8.)

12.24   EXPIRED PROTOCOLS

A PI fails to heed notices that his protocol is about to expire and fails to apply for a renewal or extension. Facing an immediate need for animals, he requests more animals and dates his request a day or two before the protocol expiration date. Theoretically, there is nothing to prevent this investigator from continuing his experiments long after the protocol covering them has expired. Although this seldom happens, IACUCs should give some thought as to how to handle this situation.

12.25   DISASTER PLANS

California has earthquakes, the Midwest has tornadoes, the South has hurricanes, and most facilities can catch fire. Because all of these disasters can have catastrophic effects on animals, should the IACUC not become a partner in all disaster plans?

12.26   USE OF ANIMALS IN PRECOLLEGE
EDUCATION

Parenthetically, the use of live animals for teaching at the grade school, middle school, and high school levels is still being debated. Although IACUCs do not enter the picture here, clear guidelines have been developed for science fairs, and these have frequently been adopted for classroom situations.

SOURCES AND SUGGESTED READING

Institute of Laboratory Animal Resources, *Guide for the Care and Use of Laboratory Animals,* National Research Council, Washington, D.C., 1996.

Schwindaman, D. F., USDA Status Report, Public responsibility in medicine and research, Spring meeting, "Animal Care and Use: Hot Zones, Gray Zones, and 'Go Slow' Zones," Boston, MA, 1996.

Silverman, J., Do pressure and prejudice influence the IACUC?, *Lab Animal,* 26(5), 23, 1997.

Carmack, B. J., and Becker, J., Staff stress, *Lab Animal,* 17(2), 21, 1988.

C. A. Pinkert, Ed., *Transgenic Animal Technology: A Laboratory Handbook,* Academic Press, San Diego, CA, 1994.

Spinelli, J. S., Changing stresses in the research community: a personal perspective, *Lab Animal,* 26(10), 41, 1997.

Danneman, P. J., Preemptive Analgesia, Presentation, American College of Laboratory Animal Medicine, 1996 Forum on Transgenic Animals and IACUC Issues, Annapolis, MD, 1996.

Wolfe, T. L., Control of Pain and Distress—The *Other* Alternative, Presentation, American College of Laboratory Animal Medicine, 1996 Forum on Transgenic Animals and IACUC Issues, Annapolis, MD, 1996.

Russell, R. J., Summary—Curbstone Session—Optimizing Use of Animal Research Facilities, Applied Research Ethics National Association Spring Meeting, Effectively Managing Animal Care and Use Programs in an Era of Diminishing Resources: Proactive Strategies, Boston, MA, 1996.

Botting, J., Dispelling myths about penicillin: the importance of using the right model, *Lab. Animal,* 26(1), 21, 1997.

International Science and Engineering Fair Operational Guidelines for Scientific Review Committees (SRCs) and Institutional Review Boards (IRBs), Science Service, Inc., Washington, D.C., 1998.

Principles and Guidelines for the Use of Animals in Precollege Education, Institute of Laboratory Animal Resources, National Research Council, National Academy Press, Washington, D.C., 1989

Acronyms and Abbreviations

AAALAC	Association for Assessment and Accreditation of Laboratory Animal Care International
AALAS	American Association for Laboratory Animal Science
ACLAM	American College of Laboratory Animal Medicine
AHA	American Heart Association
ALAT	Assistant Laboratory Animal Technician
APHIS	Animal and Plant Health Inspection Service
ARENA	Applied Research Ethics National Association
ASR	The Academy of Surgical Research
AV	Attending Veterinarian
AVMA	Animal Veterinary Medical Association
AWA	Animal Welfare Act
AWIC	Animal Welfare Information Center
CAAT	Center for Alternatives to Animal Testing
CCAC	Canadian Council on Animal Care
CEO	Chief Executive Officer
CPSC	Consumer Product Safety Commission
DEA	Drug Enforcement Administration
DVM	Doctor of Veterinary Medicine
EPA	Environmental Protection Agency
FASEB	Federation of American Societies for Experimental Biology
FDA	Food and Drug Administration
FOIA	Freedom of Information Act
Guide	*Guide for the Care and Use of Laboratory Animals*
IACUC	Institutional Animal Care and Use Committee
ILAR	Institute for Laboratory Animal Research
IO	Institutional Official
IRB	Institutional Review Board
LAT	Laboratory Animal Technician
LATG	Laboratory Animal Technologist
LAWTE	Laboratory Animal Welfare Training Exchange
LOA	Letter of Assurance
NABR	National Association for Biomedical Research
NAL	National Agricultural Library
NCRR	National Center for Research Resources
NIH	National Institutes of Health
NLM	National Library of Medicine
NRC	National Research Council
NSF	National Science Foundation

OPRR	Office of Protection from Research Risks
OSHA	Occupational Safety and Health Administration
PHS	Public Health Service
PHS Policy	The Public Health Service Policy on Humane Care and Use of Laboratory Animals
PI	Principal Investigator
PRIM&R	Public Responsibility in Medicine and Research
QA	Quality Assurance
REAC	Regulatory Enforcement and Animal Care
RVTs	Registered Veterinary Technicians
SCAW	Scientists Center for Animal Welfare
USDA	U.S. Department of Agriculture
VMD	Doctor of Veterinary Medicine

A Resources for IACUC Information

CONTENTS

A.1 PAMPHLETS

Animal Euthanasia
January 1990–November 1997
Special Reference Briefs Series No. SRB 98-01
Compiled by Michael D. Kreger
ANIMAL WELFARE INFORMATION CENTER
National Agricultural Library
10301 Baltimore Ave.
Beltsville, MD 20705-2351

A.2 AGENCIES

ANIMAL WELFARE

INFORMATION CENTER
National Agricultural Library
Beltsville, MD 20705
(301)344-3212; (301) 504-6212
The Animal Welfare Information
  Center (AWIC) of the National
  Agricultural Library (NAL) was
  established by the Animal Welfare Act.

CARE CD (Compendium of Animal
  Resources)
P.O. Box 371954
Pittsburgh, PA 15250-7954
Fax orders: (202) 512-2250
  Phone orders: (202) 512-1800

CENTER FOR ANIMALS
  AND PUBLIC POLICY
Tufts University School
  of Veterinary Medicine
200 Westboro Road
North Grafton, MA 01536
(508) 839-5302, ext. 4750

INSTITUTE OF
  LABORATORY
  ANIMAL RESOURCES
Commission on Life
  Sciences
2100 Constitution Avenue
Washington, D.C. 20418
(202) 334-2590

THE HASTINGS CENTER
255 Elm Road
Briarcliff Manor, NY 10510
(914) 762-8500

THE JOSEPH F. MORGAN
  RESEARCH FOUNDATION
P.O. Box 5002
Merivale Depot
Nepean, ON, Canada K2C 3H3
(613) 232-3260

NATIONAL LIBRARY OF MEDICINE
8600 Rockville Pike
Bethesda, MD 29892
(301) 496-3147

PUBLIC RESPONSIBILITY
  IN MEDICINE AND RESEARCH
132 Boylston Street, 4th Floor
Boston, MA 02116
(617) 423-4112

SCIENTISTS CENTER
  FOR ANIMAL WELFARE
4805 St. Elmo Avenue
Bethesda, MD 20814
(301) 654-6390

ANIMAL WELFARE INSTITUTE
P.O. Box 3650
Georgetown Station
Washington, D.C. 20007
(202) 337-2332

Applied Research Ethics
  National Association
  (ARENA)
132 Boylston Street, 4th Floor
Boston, MA 02116
(617) 423-4112

CANADIAN COUNCIL
  ON ANIMAL CARE
1000-151 Slater Street
Ottawa, ON, Canada KIP 5H3
(613) 238-4031

CENTER FOR ALTERNATIVES
  TO ANIMAL TESTING
The Johns Hopkins University
615 North Wolfe Street,
Room 1604
Baltimore, MD 20215
(410) 955-3343

B Training Resources

AALAS: American Association for Laboratory Animal Science; a professional organization for veterinarians, animal care workers, managers, and manufacturers in laboratory animal science; Mike Sondag, Executive Director, 70 Timber Creek Drive, Suite 5, Cordova, TN 38018, Phone: (901) 754-8620.

AWIC: Animal Welfare Information Center; an information center of the National Agricultural Library, established as a result of the 1985 amendment to the Animal Welfare Act; National Agricultural Library, 10301 Baltimore Avenue, Beltsville, MD 20705-2351, Phone: (301) 504-6212.

CAAT: Center for Alternatives to Animal Testing; established in 1981 to encourage and support the development of nonanimal testing methods; the Center supports grants, sponsors symposia, and publishes a variety of materials; Johns Hopkins School of Public Health, 111 Market Place, Suite 840, Baltimore, MD 21202, Phone: (410) 223-1693.

NABR: National Association for Biomedical Research; an association of biomedical facilities concerned with legislation on laboratory animal welfare and with presenting information about the benefits to human health resulting from animal experiments; Frankie Trull, Executive Director, 818 Connecticut Avenue, NW, Suite 303, Washington, D.C. 20006, Phone: (202) 857-0540.

NLM: National Library of Medicine; maintains an extensive collection of source materials and references on the basic veterinary sciences and clinical veterinary medicine with emphasis on areas closely associated with human health and health research; National Library of Medicine, Coordinator of Veterinary Affairs, Bethesda, MD 20892, Phone: (301) 496-6308.

RA!: Research America!; a group of organizations and institutions that supports animal research; Keri Sperry, Director of Communications, Suite 250, 99 Canal Center Plaza, Alexandria, VA 22314, Phone: (703) 739-2577.

SCAW: Scientists Center for Animal Welfare; a nonprofit educational organization of scientists that upholds justifiable animal research and programs to help ensure compliance with federal policies, introduction of alternatives where feasible, and sensitivity to humane issues among scientists; Lee Krulisch, Director, Golden Triangle Building One, 7833 Walter Drive, Suite 340, Greenbelt, MD 20770, Phone: (301) 345-3500.

WARDS: Working for Animals Used in Research, Drugs and Surgery; perform consulting services to inform organizations and institutions about the use of animals in research; 8150 Leesburg Pike, Suite 512, Vienna, VA 22181-2714, Phone: (703) 442-4511.

C Directory for Alternatives to Animal Testing

CONTENTS

The definition of alternatives extends to all efforts to fulfill the three R's (Russel & Burch, 1959).

1. *Reduction* of numbers of animals *(statistically significant yet not unnecessarily duplicative)*.
2. *Refinement* of procedures that decrease pain and/or distress in animals *(from psychological enrichment to appropriate use of analgesics)*.
3. *Replacement* of mammalian animals with nonanimal, nonmammalian or invertebrate species *(appropriateness of species)*.

C.1 SUGGESTED READING

Alternatives to the Use of Live Vertebrates in Biomedical Research and Testing, A bibliography with abstracts, prepared by the Toxicological and Environmental Health Information Program, Specialized Information Services, National Library of Medicine, National Institutes of Health, Bethesda, MD 20892.

C.2 PRODUCTS

(Mention of products here does not imply endorsement by either the University of California or the U.S. Department of Agriculture.)

Many CD-ROM products are available from SilverPlatter Information Company, Inc., 100 River Ridge Drive, Norwood, MA 02062; Phone: (617) 769-2599; Fax: (617) 769-8763.

For other suppliers, contact Updata Publications Inc., 1736 Westwood Boulevard, Los Angeles, CA 90024; Phone: (310) 474-5900; Fax: (310) 474-4095; Internet: gopher.updata.com; E-mail: cdrom@updata.com.

C.3   DIRECTORY

Animal Welfare Institute
P.O. Box 3650
Georgetown Station
Washington, D.C. 20007
Phone: (202) 337-2332

Association for Assessment and
  Accreditation of Laboratory Animal
  Care, International   (AAALAC)
11300 Rockville Pike
Rockville, MD 20852-3035
Phone: (301) 231-5353
Fax: (301) 231-8282
Website: http://www.aaalac.org

American Association for Laboratory
  Animal Science (AALAS)
70 Timber Creek Drive, Suite 5
Cordova, TN 38018
Phone: (901) 754-8620
Fax: (901) 753-0046
Website http://www.aalas.org

American College of Laboratory Animal
  Medicine (ACLAM)
University of Illinois, College of
  Veterinary Medicine
Division of Comparative Medicine
2001 S. Lincoln—1234 VMBSB
Urbana, IL 61801
Phone: (217) 244-1829
Fax: (217) 333-4628

American Society of Laboratory Animal
  Practitioners (ASLAP)
University of Pennsylvania
1 Blockley Hall
Philadelphia, PA 19104-6021
Phone: (215) 898-9026
Fax: (215) 898-0309

American Veterinary Medical Association
  (AVMA)
930 North Meacham Road
Schaumberg, IL 60196
Phone: (800) 248-2862
Fax: (708) 025-1329

Animal Welfare Information Center
  (AWIC) (established by the Animal
  Welfare Act)
National Agricultural Library—
  Room 301
Beltsville, MD 20705
Phone: (301) 504-5215, (301) 344-3212
Fax: (301) 504-5472
Website: http://www.nal.usda.gov/awic

Applied Research Ethics National
  Association (ARENA)
132 Boylston Street—Fourth Floor
Boston, MA 02116
Phone: (617) 423-4112
Fax: (617) 423-1185

Biological Models and Materials
  Research Program
5333 Westbard Avenue, Room 8A07
Bethesda, MD 20892
Phone: (301) 402-0630
Fax: (301) 480-2470

Canadian Council on Animal Care
151 Slater
Ottawa, ON, Canada K1P 5H3
Phone: (613) 238-4031
Fax: (613) 238-2837

Center for Animals and Public Policy
Tufts University School of Veterinary
  Medicine
200 Westboro Road
North Grafton, MA 01536
Phone: (508) 839-5302, ext. 4750
Fax: (508) 839-2953

Center for Alternatives to Animal Testing
  (CAAT)
Johns Hopkins School of Public Health
615 North Wolfe Street
Baltimore, MD 21205
Phone: (410) 955-3343
Fax: (410) 955-0258
Website:
  http://www.sph.jhu.edu/~altweb/

Center for Evaluation of Alternative
  Toxicological Methods (HIEHS)
P.O. Box 12233
Research Triangle Park, NC 27709-1233
Website:
  http://ntp-server.niehs.nih.gov/htdocs/
  ICCVAM/ICCVAM.html

Institute for Laboratory Animal
  Resources (ILAR)
National Research Council
National Academy of Sciences
2101 Constitution Avenue, NW
Washington, D.C. 20418
Phone: (202) 334-2590
Fax: (202) 334-1687

The Hastings Center
255 Elm Road
Briarcliff Manor, NY 10510
Phone: (914) 762-8500

Joseph F. Morgan Research
  Foundation
P.O. Box 5002
Merivale Depot
Nepean, ON, Canada K2C 3H3
Phone: (613) 232-3260
Fax:
Website:

National Association for Biomedical
  Research (NABR)
818 Connecticut Avenue, NW,
  Suite 303
Washington, D.C. 20006
Phone: (202) 857-0540
Fax: (202) 659-1902
Website:

National Library of Medicine
  (NLM)
8600 Rockville Pike
Bethesda, MD 29894
Phone: (800) 272-4787, (301) 496-3147
Fax: (301) 496-2809
Website:
  http://sis.nim.nih.gov/altanimals.htm

Office of Laboratory Animal Research
  (OLAR)
OER, NIH
9000 Rockville Pike
Building 1, Room 252
Bethesda, MD 20892
Website:
  http://www.sph.jhu.edu/~altweb

Office for Protection from Research
  Risks (OPRR)
Division of Animal Welfare
National Institutes of Health
Building 31, Room 5B59
Bethesda, MD 20892
Phone: (301) 498-7163
Fax: (301) 402-2803
Website.
  http://ww.nih.gov:80/grants/oprr/
  library_animal.htm

Primate Information Center
Jackie L. Pritchard, Ph.D.,
  Manager
University of Washington SJ-59
Seattle, WA 98195-7330
Phone: (206) 543-4376
Fax: (206) 685-0305
E-mail:
  pic@bart.rprc.washington.edu

Public Responsibility in Medicine and
  Research (PRIM&R)
132 Boylston Street
Boston, MA 02116
Phone: (617) 423-4112
Fax: (617) 423-1185

Scientists Center for Animal Welfare
  (SCAW)
4805 St. Elmo Avenue
Bethesda, MD 20814-4805
Phone: (301) 654-6390
Fax: (301) 907-3993
Website:
  http://www.erols.com/scaw/scaw.htm

UC Center for Animal Alternatives
School of Veterinary Medicine
University of California
Davis, CA 95616
Website: http://www.vetmed.ucdavis.edu/
  Animal_Alternatives/main.htm

C.4   DATABASES AND WEBSITES

Alternatives in Education Database:
http: //envirolink.org/arrs/avar/alted_db.htm

Altweb: http://www.sph.jhu.edu/~altweb/

BIOSIS: BIOSIS, 2100 Arch Street, Philadelphia, PA 19103-1399; Phone: (215) 587-4847, Fax: (215) 587-2016, http://www.biosis.org

DIALOG: Knight-Ridder Information, Inc., 2440 W. El Camino Real, Mountain View, CA 94040, Phone: (800) 334-2564, Fax: (650) 254-8123, E-mail: customer//www.krinfo.com

EMBASE: http://www.elsevier.com:80/ElsevierHome.html

GRATEFUL MED: contact your regional medical library at (800) 338-7657; to apply for a user code, contact the NLM MEDLARS Service Desk at (800) 648-8480

Free access to MEDLINE: http://www.nlm.nih.gov/databases/freemedl.html

NORINA: http://oslovet.veths.no/NORINA

PREX Biomedical Databases: PREX, Utrecht University, P.O. Box 80166, NL 3508 TD, Utrecht, The Netherlands, Phone: 31302533158, Fax: 31302536747, E-mail: j.d.kuiper@cc.ruu.nl or prex@pdk.dgk.ruu.nl http: //dgkp.pdk.dgk.ruu.nl/wca.dir/PREXINFO.htm

PRIMATES database: contact Jackie L. Pritchard, Ph.D., Manager, Primate Information Center, Box 357330, University of Washington, Seattle, WA 98195-7330; Phone: (206) 543-4376; Fax: (206) 685-0305; E-mail: pic@bart.rprc.washington.edu

Global Website for Alternatives to Animal Testing (in developmental stages): http://infonet.welch.jhu.edu/~caat

D Major Databases

Major databases include:

- AGRICOLA 1970 to the present

Literature citations (often with abstracts) cover veterinary medicine, laboratory animal sciences, animal welfare, and alternatives as well as agriculture and other life sciences. Sources include 1400 journals as well as textbooks, reports, monographs, theses, newsletters, professional magazines, and U.S. and foreign government publications; size: 4 million records. Produced by the National Agricultural Library, U.S. Department of Agriculture, United States.

- CAB-INTERNATIONAL DATABASES 1972 to the present

Literature citations (often with abstracts) cover veterinary science, laboratory animal science, animal welfare, animal health, animal breeding, dairy science, dairy technology, and nutrition. Sources include journals, books, serial monographs, reports, newsletters, theses, symposium proceedings, and so on; size: 800,000 records. Updated every month. Produced by CAB-International, United Kingdom.

- MEDLINE 1984 to the present

Literature citations (often with abstracts) cover the broad field of biomedical and clinical research, veterinary medicine, laboratory animal science, animal welfare, and alternatives. Sources include 3400 journals; size: 3.5 million records. Produced by the U.S. National Library of Medicine, United States.

- CSA LIFE SCIENCES 1985 to the present

Literature citations (often with abstracts) cover 20 life science disciplines from biomedical topics to viral genetics, including information on laboratory animal science. Sources include more than 5000 journals, selected books, conference reports, and U.S. patents; size: 1,074,000 records. Produced by Cambridge Scientific Abstracts, United States.

Core databases include:

- AT ALTERNATIVES circa 1920s to the present

Literature citations on alternatives to animal experiments; size: 13,000 records. Updated twice a year. Produced by Akademie für Tierschultz, Germany. Supported by National Center for Alternatives (INCA) in The Netherlands.

- BIOLOGICAL VALUES

Biological reference values of laboratory animals and hematological and clinical chemistry values with literature references and statistical parameters. This database is currently being developed; size: 7000 records. Produced by PREX Utrecht University, The Netherlands.

- BIOMEDICAL DISSERTATIONS

Biomedical academic dissertations (including abstracts) from Dutch universities; size: 3600 records. Produced by Euroscience, The Netherlands.

- BOOKS

Contents (chapter titles and bibliographic details) of 250 books on laboratory animal science; size: 6500 records. Produced by PREX, Utrecht University, The Netherlands.

- CABLINE

Index of agricultural and veterinary journals including journal title, ISSN, publisher, and country of publication; size: about 9000 records. Produced by CAB-International, United Kingdom.

- CURRENT CITATION 1995 to the present

Literature citations (without abstracts) of 11,000 journals. These are the most frequently requested journals for document delivery by the British Library; size: 2 million records. Updated every month. Produced by the British Library, United Kingdom.

- DRUG DOSAGES

Drug dosage database for nonantibiotic drugs. Contains information on 12,000 dosing regimens for more than 800 drugs. More than 4500 of the dosages provided are for anesthetic and analgesic drugs. Animals covered include all laboratory and farm animals, zoo animals, fish, amphibians, and reptiles. Corresponds to VETBASE, a PC version (see *AWIC Newsletter,* 8(1), 20, 1997). Produced by J. D. Kuiper, Ph.D., and H. J. Kuiper, Ph.D., Utrecht University, The Netherlands.

- INSIDE CONFERENCES

Citations (without abstracts but including keywords) covering conferences on a wide range of topics, including biomedical and clinical research; information includes author and title of presentation, conference title, date, and venue; size: over 2 million records. Produced by the British Library, United Kingdom.

- LABORATORY ANIMAL LITERATURE circa 1920s to the present

Literature references (including keywords) from the core journals in laboratory animal science; includes information on husbandry, genetics, origins of animal strains, techniques, veterinary care, and so on, size: 12,000 records. Produced by PREX Utrecht University, The Netherlands.

- NORINA (Norwegian Inventory of Audiovisuals)

Index of audiovisual media (including video tapes, slides) with abstract, availability, and other details; source for teaching material on laboratory animal science; size: 2700 records. Updated every year. Produced by Adrian Smith, Ph.D., and Richard Fosse, D.V.M., Norway.

- SERLINE

Index of biomedical journals with complete and abbreviated title, language, ISSN, and keywords to describe the scope of the journal; size: over 31,000 records. Updated every year. Produced by the U.S. National Library of Medicine, United States.

- STRAIN DESCRIPTION

Description of the characteristics of inbred mouse and rat strains; subjects are origin, behavior, physiology, pathology, and literature references; size: 700 records. Produced by M. F. W. Festing, Ph.D., United Kingdom.

E Where to Contact the USDA

You may contact the USDA, the Animal and Plant Health Inspection Service (APHIS), and Animal Care at the following:

Headquarters
  W. Ron DeHaven, D.V.M.
  4700 River Road, Unit 84
  Riverdale, MD 20737-1234
  Phone: (301) 734-4981
  Fax: (301) 734-4993

Eastern Region
  Elizabeth Goldentyer, D.V.M.
  2568-A Riva Road, Suite 302
  Annapolis, MD 21401
  Phone: (410) 571-8692
  Fax: (410) 224-2854

Central Region
  Walter Christensen, D.V.M.
  P.O. Box 6258
  Fort Worth Federal Center, Building 11
  Fort Worth, TX 76115
  Phone: (817) 885-6910
  Fax: (817) 885-6917

Western Region
  Robert Gibbens, D.V.M.
  9580 Micron Avenue, Suite J
  Sacramento, CA 95827
  Phone: (916) 857-6205
  Fax: (916) 857-6212

F Internet Sources of Interest to IACUCs

http://www.w3.org/hypertex/Data Sources/by Subject/Overview.html
WWW Virtual Library Main Reference

http://golgi.harvard.edu/biopages.html
WWW Virtual Library Biosciences

http://www1.mosby.com/Mosby/netvet
Mosby's Veterinary Guide to the Internet (netvet)

http://netvet.wustl.edu/biopages.html
WWW Virtual Library Veterinary Medicine

http://ss.niah.affrc.go.jp/NIAH/mirror//vetmed/vetmed.html
WWW Virtual Library Veterinary Medicine Mirror Site in Japan

http://netvet.wustl.edu/
NetVet Veterinary Resources

http://sis.nlm.nih.gov/altanimals.html
National Library of Medicine (NLM)

http://www.sph.jhu.edu/~altweb
Office of Laboratory Animal Research

http://www.vet.cornell.edu/consultant/consult.asp
Consult a Veterinarian Diagnostic Support Program

http://www.users.dircon.co.uk/~ufaw3/
Universities Federation for Animal Welfare

http://netvet.wustl.edu/e-zoo.html
The Electronic Zoo

http://vs247.cas.psu.edu/iacucsur.html
IACUCs: Celebrating 10 years of experience

http://www.nal.usda.gov/awic
IACUC and animal care bibliographies, resource guides, and bulletins

http://wwu.apa.org/science/anguide.html
APA—Guideline for Ethical Conduct In the Care and Use of Animals

gopher://gopher.vt.cdu:70/OR26406-335341m/administration/healthsafe
   /animalrespol
IACUC—Virginia Tech

http://www.uidaho.edu/research/acuc/
University of Idaho IACUC

http://clacc.uchc.edu
Animal Care Committee—University of Connecticut

http://www.ehs.ucdavis.edu/~fztilman/iahome.html
Animal Use and Care Administrative Advisory Committee (University of California, Davis)

http://www.umt.edu/research/iacuc.htm
IACUC—University of Montana

http://cpmcnet.columbia.edu/dept/icm/
CPMCNET:Institute of Comparative Medicine—Columbia University

http://www.uark.edu/admin/rsspinfo/iacuc/iacuc.html
IACUC—University of Arkansas

http://www3.umdnj.edu/~layne/vivarium.html
Vivarium Home Page, University of Medicine and Dentistry, New Jersey

http://omni.ucsb.edu/pro/acc-home.html
University of California—Santa Barbara Office of Research Animal Care Council

http://web.vet.cornell.edu/CRAR/guidelin.htm
Cornell University IACUC: New Guidelines for Animal Record Keeping

http://www.whitehouse.gov/WH/EOP/OMB/html/circulars/a021/a021.html
OMB Circular No. A-21 (Cost Principles for Educational Institutions)

http://www.aamc.org/research/primr/arena/
Applied Research Ethics National Association

http://rncc.bih.harvard.edu:80/labs/animal/animal.html
Research Administration, Animal Facility, Harvard University

http://wwwmed.stanford.edu/MedSchool/CompMed/index.html
Stanford University Department of Comparative Medicine

http://nhse.cs.rice.edu/TRAM/forms/acc.pc.html
Animal Care Committee Forms for the PC, Rice University

http://oslovet.veths.no/NORINA/NORINA—
Norwegian Inventory of Audiovisuals

http://www.usask.ca/!ladd/vet_libraris .html
Veterinary Medical Libraries Home Page

http://brise.ere.umontreal.cal~jettejp/
La Bibliotheque de Medecine Veterinaire (Universite de Montreal)

http://www.nal.usda.gov/awic/legislat/regspage.htm
USDA Animal Welfare Act

http://www.nih.gov/grants/oprr/library_animal.htm
OPRR website, from Chapter 9

http://www.aphis.usda.gov
USDA Animal and Plant Health Inspection Service

http://www.ortge.ufl.eud/iacuc/
University of Florida IACUC

http://www.aalas.org/
http://www.aalas.org/links.htm
AALAS—American Association of Laboratory Animal Science

http://phs.os.dhhs.gov/phs/phs.html
PHS—Public Health Service

http://www.ncrr.nih.gov/
NCRR—National Center for Research Resources (NIH-USA)

http://www.access.gpo.gov/su_docs/aces/aces140.html
Federal Register

gopher://gopher.legislate.com/
LEGI-SLATE Gopher Service

http://www.lib.lsu.edu/gov/fedgov.html
WWW Virtual Library: U.S. federal government agencies

http://www.cdc.gov/CDC
Centers for Disease Control

http://vetpath1.afip.mil/AFIP
Armed Forces Institute of Pathology, Department of Veterinary Pathology

http://www.aaalac.org/
AAALAC International

http://chopin.osp.uh.edu/!rocky/aclam/hdg1055.thm
ACLAM—American College of Laboratory Animal Medicine

http://www2.nas.edu/ilarhome/ILAR
Institute of Laboratory Animal Resources

http://www.nabr.org/
NABR—National Association for Biomedical Research

http://www.nap.edu/readingroom/books/labrats/
Guide for the Care and Use of Laboratory Animals (1996 edition)

http://www.aamc.org/research/primr/
PRIM&R—Public Responsibility in Medicine and Research

http://www.welch.jhu.edu/services/guides/dbs/animal.html
Searching the Journal Literature for Animal Welfare Information
(Johns Hopkins University)

http://www.outbreak.org/cgi-unreg/dynaserve.exe/index/html
Emerging disease information

http://www.ncrr.nih.gov/cost/costman/.htm
NIH Cost Analysis and Rate Setting Manual

http://cos.gdb.org/best/fed-fund.html
Federally funded research in the United States

The following resources refer to the USDA animal care regulations.

http://www.aphis.usda.gov/reac/
http://www.nal.usda.gov/awic/ legislat/regspage.htm
http://netvet.wustl.edu/awa.htm
http://netvet.wustl.edu/compmed.htm
http://netvet.wustl.edu/vetmed.htm
http://www.animal-law.org/welfact/index.html

The following Internet sites are fee-based.

http://www.dtic.mil/
Defense Technical Information Center database

http://www.frame-uk.demon.co.uk
FRAME web site for: Russell & Burch House, 96-98 North Sherwood Street,
    Nottingham, NG1 4EE, United Kingdom

G Associations and Related Organizations

Allied Trade Association (ATA)
Deborah A. Benner
(215) 855-1040
Fax: (215) 362-8410
E-mail: brownp@31b4.nic.nih.gov

American Animal Hospital Association
P.O. Box 150899
Denver, CO 80215-08899
(303) 986-2800

American Association for Laboratory
Animal Science (AALAS)
70 Timber Creek Drive
Cordova, TN 38018
(901) 754-8620

American Association of Human–
Animal Bond Veterinarians
University of Florida
College of Veterinary Medicine
Box 100136
Gainesville, FL 32610
(352) 392-4700, ext. 4024

American Association of Industrial
Veterinarians
P.O. Box 488
Oskaloosa, KS 66066-0488
(913) 863-2389

American Association of Laboratory
Animal Practitioners
University of Texas Medical School
6431 Fannin Street, Room 1132
Houston, TX 77030
(713) 500-7542

American Board of Veterinary
Toxicology
University of Pennsylvania
School of Veterinary Medicine
New Bolton Center
382 W. Street Road
Kennet Square, PA 19348
(610) 444-5800, ext. 2217

American College of Laboratory Animal
Medicine (ACLAM)
200 Summerwinds Drive
Cary, NC 27511
(919) 859-5985

American College of Veterinary
Anesthesiologists
Colorado State University
Department of Clinical Sciences
Fort Collins, CO 80523
(970) 491-0346

American College of Veterinary
Pathologists
875 Kings Highway, Suite 200
Woodbury, NJ 08096
(609) 348-7784

American College of Zoological
Medicine
White Oak Conservation Center
726 Owens Road
Yulee, FL 32097
(904) 225-3387

American Committee on Laboratory
  Animal Disease (ACLAD)
John D. Strandberg
(410) 955-3273
Fax: (410) 550-5068
E-mail:
  jstrand@welchlink.welch.jhu.edu

American Fisheries Society
5410 Grosvenor Lane, Suite 110
Bethesda, MD 20814
(301) 897-8616

Americans for Medical
  Progress (AMP)
421 King Street, Suite 401
Alexandria, VA 22314

American Society of Animal Science
111 North Dunlop Avenue
Savoy, IL 61874
(217) 356-3182

American Veterinary Distributors
  Association
106 W. 11th Street, Suite 1200
Kansas City, MO 64105
(816) 221-5909

American Veterinary Medical
  Association (AVMA)
1931 N. Meacham Road, Suite 100
Schaumberg, IL 60173-4360
(847) 925-8070

Animal Protection Institute of America
P.O. Box 22505
Sacramento, CA 95822
(916) 731-5521

Animal Transportation Association
P.O. Box 60564, AMS
Houston, TX 77205
(281) 443-4595

Animal Welfare Institute
P.O. Box 3650
Washington, D.C. 20007
(202) 337-2332

Association of Assessment and
  Accreditation of Laboratory Animal
  Care, International (AAALAC,
  International)
11300 Rockville Pike, Suite 1211
Rockville, MD 20815
(301) 231-5353

Association for Gnotobiotics
Patricia M. Bealmear
(716) 655-1680
Fax: (716) 655-1680

Association of Primate Veterinarians
9200 Leesburg Pike
Vienna, VA 22182
(703) 759-7880, ext. 5390

Association of Reptilian and Amphibian
  Veterinarians
Box 605
Chester Heights, PA 19017
(610) 358-9530

Association of Veterinary Technician
  Educators
Dr. Peter Bill
Veterinary Technology
Lynn Hall
Purdue University
West Lafayette, IN 47907
(765) 494-8639

Canadian Association for Laboratory
  Animal Science (CALAS)
Donald McKay
(403) 429-5193
Fax: (403) 492-7257
E-mail: dmckay@gpu.srv.ualberta.ca

H Guidelines for Blood Sample Withdrawal

Katy Wilson, D.V.M.

The purpose of these guidelines is:

1. To provide researchers with the necessary information to determine the single maximum blood withdrawal and also multiple blood sample withdrawals on a weekly basis. These guidelines apply to healthy, adult animals. The use of immature or debilitated animals requires consultation with the veterinary staff.
2. To give IACUC members, during protocol reviews, figures that represent reasonable and acceptable amounts of blood that may be withdrawn.

Excessive blood volume withdrawal can cause increases in cortisol, decreases in prolactin, blood pressure, and tissue/organ perfusion, as well as lactic acidosis, tachycardia, dyspnea, gastrointestinal ulceration, organ failure, and death. Less severe consequences to chronic low-level blood loss such as folic acid/iron deficiency and anemia can also result. Fluids, plasma, resuspended red cells, or iron/vitamin B replacement therapies should be considered when drafting a sampling schedule. For studies requiring multiple blood sampling, the same site should not be used for two consecutive withdrawals.

Total Blood Volume

Species	ml/kg of Body Weight
Mouse	90
Rat	64 (58–70)*
Hamster	87
Guinea Pig	75 (67–92)*
Rabbit	56 (44–70)*
Dog	86
Monkey	77
Swine	75

* Higher values in the range apply to younger, lighter weight animals.

- Recommended maximum cumulative withdrawal is less than or equal to 8 percent of blood volume per week.

  Examples
  Rat: 250 g 0.25 kg $\times$ 70 ml/kg $\times$ 0.08 (8%) = 1.4 ml of blood per week.
  Dog: 8 kg 8 kg $\times$ 86 ml/kg $\times$ 0.08 (8%) = 55 ml of blood per week.

- A single maximum withdrawal should be less than or equal to 10 to 15 percent of blood volume with a 30-day recovery period.
- Animals undergoing the maximum volume blood withdrawal should be evaluated for anemia or iron deficiency before being placed on another study.

REFERENCES

1. McGuill, M. W. and Rowan, A. N., Biological effects of blood loss, *ILAR J.,* 31(4), 5, 1989.
2. Morton, D. B., et al., Removal of blood from laboratory mammals, *Lab. Anim.,* 27, 1, 1993.

I Volume Guidelines for Compound Administration

Victor Lukas, D.V.M.

The purpose of these guidelines is:

1. To provide researchers with *maximum* daily volumes of fluids or compounds that may be administered to animals. These guidelines apply for healthy, adult animals. When immature or debilitated animals are used, the veterinary staff must be consulted.

2. To give IACUC members, during protocol reviews, figures that represent reasonable and acceptable amounts of fluids or compounds that may be administered.

Volumes represented in ml/kg of body weight*

Species	Oral	Intravenous	Intraperitoneal	Subcutaneous	Intramuscular
Mouse	20.0	20.0	20.0	20.0	3.0
Rat	20.0[a]	10.0[b]	20.0[c]	20.0	1.0[d]
Hamster	20.0	10.0	20.0	20.0	1.0
Guinea Pig	20.0[a]	10.0[b]	10.0[c]	20.0	1.0[d]
Rabbit	10.0	10.0	10.0	10.0	0.5
Dog	10.0	10.0	5.0	5.0	0.5[e]
Monkey	10.0	10.0	5.0	5.0	0.5[e]
Swine	10.0	10.0	5.0	3.0	0.5[f]

Route of administration

* Multiply the appropriate number above times the animal's body weight in kg to obtain the maximum volume of administration.

The following limits supersede the maximum limits when dosing heavier animals:

[a] The maximum single oral dose for a rat or a guinea pig is 5.0 ml for animals greater than 0.25 kg.

[b] The maximum single IV dose for a rat or a guinea pig is 2.5 ml for animals greater than 0.25 kg.

[c] The maximum single IP dose for a rat is 5.0 ml for animals greater than 0.25 kg.

[d] The maximum single IM dose for a rat or a guinea pig is 0.5 ml for animals greater than 0.50 kg.

[e] The maximum single IM dose for a dog or a monkey is 3.0 ml for animals greater than 6.0 kg.

[f] The maximum single IM dose for swine is 5.0 ml for animals greater than 10.0 kg.

Administration of excessive dose volumes may produce pain, excitement, altered physiological parameters (e.g., serum electrolyte imbalance, increased blood pressure, increased respiratory rate, etc.), and cause abnormal compound absorption. A large intramuscular injection into a small muscle mass may force the dose into fascial planes and subcutaneous tissues that may accelerate lymphatic drainage and may also cause pressure necrosis or nerve damage. For parenteral routes of administration (a route other than oral), it may be less irritating to administer the dose halved in two separate locations. For studies requiring repeated parenteral dosing, the same site should not be used for two consecutive administrations.

In addition to volume of administration, one must also consider the character of the solution. Known irritants such as Freund's adjuvant should be delivered according to specific guidelines/protocols. Solutions above pH 8.0 and below pH 4.5 should be diluted or buffered even if this means exceeding guidelines, provided that veterinary and IACUC approvals have been obtained. One must consider any possible affects attributable to the vehicle alone (e.g., DMSO and polyethylene glycol, etc.)

The maximum intradermal dose for all species is 0.05–0.10 ml/site. Volumes listed previously are for maximum daily cumulative administrations.

REFERENCES

1. Harkness, J. E. and Wagner, J. E., *The Biology and Medicine of Rabbits and Rodents*, 4th ed., Williams & Wilkins, 1995.
2. Foster, H. L., Small, J. D., and Fox, J. G., *The Mouse in Biomedical Research*, Vol. III, Academic Press, 1983. Bourne, G. H., Ed., *The Rhesus Monkey*, Vol. I, Academic Press, 1975.
3. Gay, W. I., Ed., *Methods of Animal Experimentation*, Vol. I, Academic Press, 1965.
4. Hull, R. M., Guideline limit volumes for dosing animals in the preclinical stage of safety evaluation, *Human and Exptl Tox*, 14, 305, 1995.

J Euthanasia Guidelines

The following notes refer to procedures to be used in methods of euthanasia by species:

1. Abbreviations:

    A means acceptable. Acceptable methods are recommended. Scientific justification for acceptable methods of euthanasia is not required in the Application to Use Vertebrate Animals in Research, Testing, or Instruction (Form 8225).

    CA means conditionally acceptable. Other methods are preferred. Scientific or other justification for conditionally acceptable methods of euthanasia is required in the Application to Use Vertebrate Animals in Research, Testing, or Instruction (Form 8225).

    U means unacceptable without justification. The selection of any of these methods is strongly discouraged. However, there may be unusual circumstances that may lead an investigator to choose an unacceptable method. If you must use an unacceptable method, scientific or other justification is required in Form 8225 and the use must be approved by the University Committee on Use and Care of Animals.

    For additional information on any method of euthanasia, request a copy of the Report of the AVMA Panel on Euthanasia. [*JAVMA*, 202(2), 229, 1993].

2. Intravenous sodium pentabarbital at dosages of 85 to 200 mg/kg is recommended for euthanasia of most species. Rats and mice may require higher dosages (150 to 220 mg/kg) than other species. Sodium secobarbital at dosages of 88 mg/kg also may be used. Intraperitoneal injection may be used in situations wherein this approach would cause less distress than intravenous injection.

3. In decreasing order of preference: halothane, enflurane, isoflurane, methoxyflurane or ether. Although ether is effective, it must be used with care because it is flammable and explosive, and for safe use requires special precautions. Signs indicating that ether is present or in use should be posted conspicuously. To avoid explosions, the carcasses of animals euthanized with ether should be stored in explosion-safe refrigerators or freezers after the ether has volatilized. Then the carcasses may be incinerated.

4. Although acceptable, inhalant anesthetics are generally not used in these species because of cost and difficulty of administration.

University of Michigan—Methods of Euthanasia by Species

METHOD[1]	Amphibians	Birds	Cats	Dogs	Fish	Horses
			Species			
Barbiturates	A[2]	A[2]	A[2]	A[2]	A[2]	A[2]
Inhalant anesthetics[3]	A	A	A	A	U	A[4]
Carbon dioxide	A[5]	A[5]	CA[5]	CA[5]	U	U
Carbon monoxide	A[6]	A[6]	A[6]	A[6]	A[6]	U
Microwave irradiation	U	U	U	U	U	U
Tricaine methanesulfonate	A[8]	U	U	U	A[8]	U
Benzocaine	A[9]	U	U	U	A[9]	U
Cervical dislocation	U	CA	U	U	U	U
Decapitation	CA[11]	CA	U	U	CA	U
Chloral hydrate	U	U	U	U	U	CA[12]
Penetrating captive bolt	CA	U	U	CA	U	CA
Gunshot	CA	U	U	U	U	CA
Electrocution	U	U	U	CA[13]	U	CA[13]
Pithing	CA[14]	U	U	U	U	U
Nitrogen, argon	U	CA	CA	CA	U	U
Nitrous oxide	U	U	U	U	U	U
Exsanguination[13]	U	U	U	U	U	U
Stunning[16]	U	U	U	U	U	U
Chloroform[17]	U	U	U	U	U	U
Air embolism[13]	U	U	U	U	U	U
Rapid freezing[13]	U	U	U	U	U	U
Nicotine[13]	U	U	U	U	U	U
Magnesium sulfate[13]	U	U	U	U	U	U
Potassium chloride[13]	U	U	U	U	U	U
Strychnine[13]	U	U	U	U	U	U
Neuromuscular blocking (curariform) agents	U	U	U	U	U	U

Note: Table courtesy of Howard G. Rush, D.V.M., Diplomate A.C.L.A.M.

5. Compressed carbon dioxide gas in cylinders is preferred. Flow rate should be 20 percent of chamber vol/min and chamber should be pre-filled to a CO_2 concentration of 70 percent or more before animals are placed in the chamber. If dry ice is used, freezing or chilling of animals must be prevented. Larger animals, such as rabbits, cats, and swine, appear to be more distressed by CO_2 euthanasia; therefore, other methods of euthanasia are preferable.

6. Use compressed carbon monoxide gas. Special procedures must be used.

7. For use with small laboratory rodents only. Specially designed equipment must be used.

METHOD[1]	Monkeys	Rabbits	Reptiles	Rodents and Other Small Animals	Ruminants	Swine
Barbiturates	A[2]	A[2]	A[2]	A[2]	A[2]	A[2]
Inhalant anesthetics[3]	A	A	A	A	A[4]	A[4]
Carbon dioxide	CA	CA[5]	A[5]	A[5]	U	CA[5]
Carbon monoxide	CA[6]	A[6]	A[6]	A[6]	U	CA[6]
Microwave irradiation	U	U	U	A[7]	U	U
Tricaine methanesulfonat	U	U	U	U	U	U
Benzocaine	U	U	U	U	U	U
Cervical dislocation	U	CA[10]	U	CA[10]	U	U
Decapitation	U	CA	CA[11]	CA	U	U
Chloral hydrate	U	U	U	U	CA[12]	CA[12]
Penetrating captive bolt	U	CA	CA	U	CA	CA
Gunshot	U	U	CA	U	CA	CA
Electrocution	U	U	U	U	CA[13]	CA[13]
Pithing	U	U	CA[14]	U	U	U
Nitrogen, argon	CA	CA	U	CA[15]	U	U
Nitrous oxide	U	U	U	U	U	U
Exsanguination[13]	U	U	U	U	U	U
Stunning[16]U	U	U	U	U	U	
Chloroform[17]U	U	U	U	U	U	
Air embolism[13]U	U	U	U	U	U	
Rapid freezing[13]U	U	U	U	U	U	
Nicotine[13]U	U	U	U	U	U	
Magnesium sulfate[13]U	U	U	U	U	U	
Potassium chloride[13]U	U	U	U	U	U	
Strychnine[13]U	U	U	U	U	U	
Neuromuscular blocking (curariform) agents	U	U	U	U	U	U

8. Fish and amphibians may be euthanized by immersion in a tank containing tricaine methanesulfonate at a concentration of 100 to 200 mg/l of water for 10 to 20 min.
9. Fish and amphibians may be euthanized by immersion in a tank containing benzocaine at a concentration of 100 to 150 mg/l of water for 10 to 20 min.
10. Manual cervical dislocation is conditionally acceptable in mice and rats weighing less than 200 g and rabbits weighing less than 1 kg. Cervical dislocation may be performed on larger rats and rabbits manually by an individual with demonstrated proficiency or if a mechanical dislocater is utilized.

11. In amphibians and reptiles, decapitation should be followed by pithing both the brain and spinal cord.

12. Horses, ruminants, and swine may be euthanized with chloral hydrate at dosages of 900 mg/kg intravenously. Sedate animal first and then give chloral hydrate intravenously.

13. This method is unacceptable as the sole method of euthanasia. However, if animals are first anesthetized or rendered unconscious by other means, this method may then be used.

14. May be used as sole method of euthanasia in species such as frogs with anatomic features that facilitate easy access to the central nervous system. In these species, both the brain and spinal cord must be pithed (i.e., double pithing). In all other species of amphibians and reptiles, pithing should be followed by decapitation.

15. When euthanizing rats, the oxygen concentration must be less than 2 percent and the animal must be heavily sedated or anesthetized.

16. Stunning is unacceptable as a sole method of euthanasia. If performed properly, stunning will produce unconsciousness but must be followed by a method to ensure the animal's death (e.g., pharmacologic agents or decapitation).

17. Chloroform is unacceptable for euthanasia. It is a known hepatotoxin and suspected carcinogen and is considered hazardous to humans.

REFERENCE

Rush, H. G., Interpretive summary of the report of the AVMA panel on euthanasia, *Contemp. Top. Lab. Anim. Sci.,* 35(2), 42, 1996.

Index

A

AAALAC, see Association for Assessment and Accreditation of Laboratory Animal Care International

AALAS, see American Association for Laboratory Animal Science

Absenteeism, 9

Academia, IACUC issues in, 33–48
  animal research at other institutions, 42–43
  assurance of protocol adherence, 43–45
    conducting investigation, 44
    filing complaint with IACUC, 43–44
    investigation of allegations, 44
    investigative findings, 44–45
    protocol noncompliance, 43
  compensation for service, 46
  establishment of satellite facilities, 42
  external review, 46
  funding sources and deadlines, 39
  IACUC membership, 35–37
  interactiveness of IACUC, 37
  principal investigator on protocol, 40
  requirements for protocol review, 39–40
  role of IACUC, 34–35
  scientific merit, 40–41
  size and diversity of research program, 37–38
  sunshine laws, 45–46
  use of animals for teaching, 41–42
  use of hazardous agents, 41

Academic institutions, receiving state funding, 45

Academy of Surgical Research (ASR), 88

Acetaminophen, 121

ACLAM, see American College of Laboratory Animal Medicine

Acronyms and abbreviations, 163–164

Administrations/nonsurgical procedures, experimental, 53

Agricultural research, 37

AHA, see American Heart Association

ALAT, see Assistant Laboratory Animal Technician

Allegations, investigation of, 44

Alternatives, literature search for, 139–152
  defining alternatives, 140
  how to search for alternatives, 142–150

describing protocol, 143–144
  designing search strategy, 144–145
  documenting alternatives search and writing narrative, 150
  executing and evaluating search, 149–150
  selecting databases, 145–149
  legislation, 140–141
  search benefits, 142
  sources and suggested reading, 151–152
  time and money, 151

American Association for Laboratory Animal Science (AALAS), 88, 103

American Cancer Society, 73

American College of Laboratory Animal Medicine (ACLAM), 92, 154

American Heart Association (AHA), 39

Analgesic
  management, gold standard of, 125
  therapy, 120, 124

Anemia, profound, 128

Anesthesia, 42, 54

Anesthesiologists, 37

Anesthetic therapy, 124

Animal(s)
  care
    responsibility for, 107
    staffs, communications between scientific and, 132
  facility
    general conditions of, 104
    semiannual inspection report form, 64
  genetically-altered, 117
  limits notice, 61
  monitoring, 137
  research ethics boards, 1
  rooms, 105
  support areas, 105
  testing, directory for alternatives to, 169–172
  unconscious, 122

Animal Care Policies, 140

Animal and Plant Health Inspection Services (APHIS), 7, 78, 141

Animal Welfare Act (AWA), 1, 18, 67, 100
  changes in field of laboratory science since, 85
  directives, 156
  1985 amendments to, 139
  regulations, 20, 103, 107